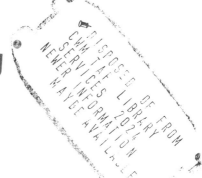

Things they don't teach you at medical school but which you will need to know to survive as a doctor are explained in *How To Do It*. The experts who wrote it learnt from experience: you can learn from this book.

In response to readers' enthusiasm it is now reprinted as *How to Do It: Volume 1*. A new compendium of essential know how, *How To Do It: Volume 2* will be published in autumn 1987.

HOW TO DO IT
Volume 1

Second edition

Articles from the *British Medical Journal*

Published by the British Medical Association
Tavistock Square, London WC1H 9JR

© British Medical Journal 1985

First published 1979
Second Impression 1980
Third Impression 1982
Fourth Impression 1983
Second Edition 1985
Second Impression 1987
Third Impression 1988
Fourth Impression 1990
Fifth Impression 1991
Sixth Impression 1993

British Library Cataloguing in Publication Data
How to do it——2nd ed.
  1. Communication in medicine
  I. British Medical Journal
  610.69'6   R118

ISBN 0-7279-0186-9

Printed and bound in Great Britain by
Latimer Trend & Company Ltd, Plymouth

Preface
to the second edition

In their early years just before and after graduation doctors face a series of unnerving and sometimes unpleasant experiences—clinical examinations and vivas, applying for a job or a research grant, and appearing before committees. No sooner have those miseries faded into the past than a whole new range of testing experiences begins—sitting on committees, acting as a referee or an examiner, or appearing in court. Rarely is anyone taught how to cope with, let alone excel at, these occasions. The original chapters in the first edition of *How to Do It* proved a useful guide to many of the potentially embarrassing set pieces that a doctor has to face. These original chapters have now been updated and expanded, and we have added several more. Some of these deal simply with tasks not included in the first edition—such as assessing a job and dealing with a publisher—while others—such as choosing a computer, flying, and holding a press conference—cover new challenges that have become more prominent in recent years.

STEPHEN LOCK
Editor
British Medical Journal

Contents

Organise an international medical meeting

IAN CAPPERAULD, A I S MACPHERSON

I: Committees and budgets

At some time in his professional career a doctor may be concerned with organising a medical meeting. Meetings range from large international ones to small local gatherings, but the principles for organising all of them are the same. We propose to state these principles, to expand on topics that are often alien to the medical mind, and to point out some of the pitfalls that may trap the unwary and uninitiated. The principles are simple, and some of the things we say will seem obvious, but the obvious is often overlooked merely because it is simple. We shall be discussing committees, budgets, scientific and social programmes, registration, and other aspects of medical meetings.

The committee

The organising committee must be carefully chosen by the chairman. This working group of people will have various tasks allotted to them, many of which will be time-consuming. It is important, therefore, to allot duties to suitable individual members. If one member of the committee flies round the world every week it would be disastrous to give him a task that demands his frequent presence. Similarly, you should think carefully about giving some jobs to the young who have energy, and others to the mature who have tact. Each member of the organising committee should chair a subcommittee to co-ordinate the main activities.

An important point in choosing the organising committee or some of the subcommittee members is to include lay people. Obtaining the help of someone in local government will smooth the path to official receptions, while the city manager or one of his senior colleagues on the committee will produce facilities and services that are invaluable to the meeting. Similarly, including a lay member who knows about finance and budgeting is imperative.

If a trade exhibition is to be held, the help of someone in the pharmaceutical industry will keep that side of the meeting under control and add to the income. The chairman should appoint subcommittees for the following (with a member of the organising committee in charge): scientific programme; social programme; finance and budgeting; audiovisual aids; ladies' programme; publicity, advertising, and trade exhibition; and transport and hotel accommodation.

The organising committee should give a definite remit to the sub-committees, which should report to the main organising committee formally at the mian monthly meeting. It is perhaps obvious, but minutes of all these meetings should be kept, and outstanding actions and promises not carried out rectified immediately by the chairman. Your organising committee should be like the board of a company, whose sole business is to run a successful meeting, ideally at a profit—but certainly not at a loss.

Financial aspects of meetings

Many doctors take fright at the words "finance" and "budget". These aspects, however, are becoming more and more important for a successful meeting, especially as costs rise. Our object is not to tell you how to raise money or what to do with it, but rather to guide you towards good management of your financial affairs. When faced with a medical meeting you must ask yourselves, "can we afford it?" and, if the answer is yes, "How can we organise the financial resources to make the meeting excellent?"

The money side of a meeting should be regarded in the same way that a housewife looks at her housekeeping. She knows how much the goods are in the shops and she knows how much money she has in her purse. By wise buying and shopping around she gets value for her money. She, in fact, works out the household budget.

Making up a budget

A budget is simply a plan of action expressed in money. Essentially, the budget should state how much money is going to be spent and how much money is going to be brought in. Indeed, such an exercise can produce only three results: the meeting will make a profit, will break even, or will incur a loss. Judicial surgical intervention by making certain cuts in the budget can convert a loss to a break even, or a break even to a profit. The first responsibility of any committee is to construct a budget since all other aspects of the meeting are dependent on this.

Cash in

The various sources of money at a medical meeting are direct registration fees; donations; and trade exhibition. Of these, only direct registration fees are completely under the control of the organising committee. Charge too much and you will dissuade many from attending. Charge too little and you may incur a loss. To be certain of viability, therefore, at least 60% of your total income should come from this source. How can you forecast how many people will attend the meeting? Past history helps, together with national or current international financial climates. It is important to remember that what may appear to be an excessively high registration fee for someone in Britain may be average or even cheap for someone abroad. In many countries registration fees are tax deductable by the medical man attending the meeting and this should be considered when calculating registration fees. The proportion of overseas to home delegates, therefore, could influence the setting of the registration fee.

Donations may be classified as coming from internal or external sources. Internal sources come from the cash reserves of the initiating society or from local university or college sources. External sources consist of local government support from city or town councils, and perhaps even central Government if the meeting merits such funding. Donations may also come from local industry, which may or may not be allied to medicine, or from industry allied to the theme of the meeting, perhaps even from abroad. You should remember that donations in kind can be just as useful as a monetary donation. Providing a reception, for example, relieves the committee and the participants of cash transfers. Also important in saving money is waiving fees for the hire of a building or a lecture theatre.

The income from a well-organised trade exhibition can contribute substantially to a successful meeting, and we give details of its organisation below. Participation by the drug industry, however, requires the courtesy of attendance by the delegates at some time during the course of the meeting, and this is not always arranged. It is a paradox that as more demands are made on the pharmaceutical industry to give support, fewer and fewer delegates appear to be attending exhibitions.

Cash out

Services, buildings, people, and commodities have to be paid for. The expenditure side of the cash budget is readily controllable. The committee can set the amount of money that they are prepared

3

to spend on certain parts of the meeting. A simple illustrative example is the entertainment laid on for the delegates. The committee may decide to be lavish, or austere. Nevertheless, when the budget is complete, the sum put in for entertainment may be increased to make thrifty entertainment pleasurable and lavish entertainment cut to make it allowable—or legal.

The same budget illustrated in the table is taken from an article[1] describing the financial aspects of a large international meeting and lists the income and expenditure of that meeting. The figure obtained from that particular meeting for registration fees came to 65% of the total income; there was a surplus or profit of $16 \cdot 7\%$.

Construction of budget

Responsibility for constructing the budget is a whole committee effort. Each member or chairman of a subcommittee group should

Income	£	Expenditure	£
Registration fees:		Salaries	15·6
Members and temporary		Office equipment	0·8
members	54·2	Telephones	1·4
Guests of members ..	10·8	Postage and freight	1·0
Trade exhibition	23·2	Stationery	0·8
Donations	0·4	Insurances	0·9
Banquet	8·2	Expenses of setting up registration offices	1·3
Bank interest	1·9		
Advertising	1·2	Expenses of setting up special	
Sundry income	0·1	office	0·4
		Staff travel	0·3
		Sundry expenses	0·4
		Input VAT not recovered ..	0·9
		Sign printing	0·9
		Printing in total	9·0
		Translation	16·6
		Rents and services	6·8
		Trade exhibition	6·2
		Briefcases and badges ..	0·8
		Transport for delegates ..	0·8
		Banquet	7·6
		Ladies' social club	0·7
		Audit fee	0·8
		Entertainment	2·2
		Commemorative envelopes ..	0·3
		VIP expenses	2·0
		Hotel bookings not taken up ..	4·8
Total	100·0	Total	83·3
		Surplus or profit	16·7

4

be able to forecast the money needed at least for his own part of the scheme. Start with the list of sums that you will have to pay out. Remember that costs in a budget may be fixed or variable. Fixed means that, whether one person or a hundred turn up, the amount to be spent for that service is the same. Good examples of fixed costs are the hire of the lecture theatre, the projectionist's fee, translation facilities, telephone installation, and insurance. Variable costs depend on the number of people attending and include such things as meals, entertainment, and certain printing costs. It is extremely difficult to be dogmatic in describing fixed and variable costs because some services contain an element of both. Nevertheless, if you stick to the principle of thinking in terms of fixed and variable costs you will avoid the trap of preparing a budget where most of the expenditure is committed to fixed costs.

Having obtained the first estimate of expenditure on the budget, increase this figure by $10–15\%$ to take into account the inflation that is likely to occur between the planning and the date of the meeting. Given that at least 60% of your income will come from registration fees you can work this out thus:

$$\text{Registration fee} = \frac{\text{total cost} + 10\%}{\text{No attending}} \times \frac{60}{100}$$

If the figure obtained is astronomical you will have to look again at the expenditure side of the budget and cut it until you reach a tolerable level for the registration fee. If such a figure cannot be decided early on, the financial aspect of the meeting spells disaster. Remember that the figures supplied are only guestimates, and the sooner accurate estimates are obtained the better the budget will be. Indeed, the decision of "go" or "no-go" in a meeting can be worked out rapidly by using this formula. When a registration fee has been fixed for years you should be able to obtain an indication of viability by changing the figures in the given formula.

With regard to the income side of the budget, the forecasted number of people attending needs to be accurate to calculate what, in effect, is 60% of your total income. You can relieve this headache by fixing the number of people allowed to attend; this simplifies the budget considerably but does not always lead to a successful meeting. If the attendance is not fixed the income from 100% attendance on as accurate a forecast as possible can be calculated. Similarly, the income from 90% and 80% attendance can be calculated, hence giving you some idea of the money available which should be balanced by making cuts on the expenditure side. In the early stages, the budget should be fluid and capable of being chopped and changed until a definite plan of action is decided. The final income and expenditure statement

5

after the meeting should only confirm the budget. It should be like an x-ray film confirming a previously clinically diagnosed condition.

As we have said, repeated revision of the budget is necessary. It should be brought up to date monthly by the full committee, so that any disasters that are beginning to show up are avoided, or at least ameliorated. The weekly meeting allows pruning of the expenditure if income is not up to forecast or adding a refinement to the programme if the income is above budget. Allowances must be made for insurance in case the meeting has to be cancelled because of airline strikes, hotel strikes, or natural disasters that could affect the meeting. The committee should be prepared to pay up to 1% of the total cost of the meeting to get such cover.

One way money may be lost is in misunderstanding whose travel expenses and whose hotel bills are going to be paid by the meeting. The committee should define these invited guests, and include their expenses in the budget. Beware of the invited guest who always has caviar and champagne for breakfast and charges it on his hotel bill. Unexpected bills are always sent in—for example, the florist has to be paid for flower arrangements at the official opening and at the banquet. Someone may decide that microphones at the banquet would be useful, and forget that this has to be paid for. Buses ordered and not used have to be paid for, as have staff who stay on because a function overruns. Telephone accounts may come in long after the meeting and often more telephones are laid on or used than have been allowed for. Beware of the individual who asks to use the official telephone and who speaks for half-an-hour at a time with New York, Tokyo, or Sydney, without reversing the charges. Often a guaranteed income is given on bar and coffee takings, and, if this is not achieved, it will be necessary to make up that deficit to the vendor.

In meetings in the UK the introduction of "value added tax" has added problems for the accountant. Certain items are subject to VAT and may be reclaimed, while sometimes VAT is payable but not reclaimable. Even corporation tax may rear its ugly head in certain circumstances. When the committee has to be concerned with VAT and corporation tax, professional help is necessary. When the time comes to pay bills, especially when they are large, you should ask whether a discount is available if you settle these accounts quickly.

Trade exhibition

When organising a conference, an important question for the committee must be whether or not to have a trade exhibition. The

6

two main benefits are firstly that it can be a useful source of money to add to the budget income, and secondly that delegates can apprise themselves of a wide range of information about many different products in a convenient and speedy way. Communication with the company representatives can solve problems and queries. If you decide to have a trade exhibition, certain conditions are essential for success:

(1) Committee and delegates alike must acknowledge its value and relevance by according courtesy and attention to the exhibitors and their displays.

(2) The exhibition space should be an integral part of the conference area, immediately adjacent to the lecture theatre, seminar rooms, or both, and large enough for its purpose.

(3) Morning coffee and afternoon tea, at least, and preferably lunch as well must be served in the exhibition area, which normally should also have registration facilities.

The organisation of the trade exhibition may be handed over to a company whose professional business it is to run exhibitions, in which case the "profit" from the exhibition will largely accrue to that company; or the committee may invite one of the exhibiting companies to organise the exhibition on behalf of the conference, for which only the expenses of the organiser will be charged and hence a bigger "profit" will go to the meeting.

To decide who is to run an exhibition, the committee must consider both the objectives of the conference and its scale. You will find it a considerable advantage to make the exhibition organiser an ex officio member of the conference committee, because this encourages closer liaison and friendly working partnership.

When the organiser has been appointed, the committee should agree estimated financial figures with him. These will include such factors as the number of exhibitors who may be safely accommodated in the space available for the exhibition, and also the charge for a square metre of exhibition space. The committee should also, if possible, provide the organiser with lists of potential exhibitors to be invited. Beyond that, they should allow him complete autonomy, subject to periodical reports on progress at meetings of the committee (hence the advantage of his membership).

It is well to remember that a conference of any kind is a business occasion and all associated arrangements must be conducted in a business-like manner. This applies equally to the trade exhibition. While the exhibition organiser will deal with detailed arrangements, the committee should be aware of the main matters to be taken care of. These may be summarised as follows:

7

(1) *Space available*—Number of stands which can safely be accommodated; and need for adequate gangways to allow stands to be seen and to meet first safety regulations.

(2) *Costs*—Costs incurred in mounting an exhibition are the rental of space, hire of furnishings and equipment, installation of temporary electric supply, electricity, and cleaning. These direct costs must be adequately covered by exhibition charges. In addition, participating companies will have their own costs covering stands, publications, samples, travel, accommodation, and salaries. The charge to the exhibitors, therefore, must be carefully worked out so that the direct costs do not exceed the total income from the sale of the exhibition space.

(3) *Timing*—Company staff who man exhibition stands will spend the greater part of any day hanging about. It is vital, therefore, to ensure that the length of time the exhibition is on display is related closely to the nature of the conference and the number of delegates. Far better to have a two-day exposure in the middle of a week's conference, than to expect exhibitors to stand around for days on end without a customer. One must also remember to allow time for setting up and dismantling.

(4) *Exhibition area*—Access for stands and equipment for display must be practical. Electricity supply must be adequate. Water supply and drainage may be necessary. Storage space for exhibitors' material before, during, and after an exhibition is essential. Security measures are often required so that valuable equipment is not stolen or broken.

(5) *Exhibition organiser*—He must be given authority to do his job—and be left to do it. All matters relating to the exhibition must be channelled through him. He will collect and pay out all exhibition money, handing over at the end of the operation a net sum with an audited statement of income and expenditure, with the hope of producing a reasonable profit to the meeting to offset some of the outgoing expenditure.

Conclusion

The problems of running a large international meeting are legion and here we have attempted to outline only some of the main financial aspects. The keys to success are accurate forecasting and tight budget control, coupled with a good accountant and a hard-working committee, meeting frequently, led by an understanding chairman. The final income and expenditure statement should only confirm the budget previously made. No one should be surprised, therefore, at the profit—or the loss.

II: Scientific programme

Responsibility for arranging the scientific programme should be given to one member of the organising committee, with powers to appoint his own programme subcommittee. Each member of this subcommittee must accept a specific job. The task of the scientific programme sub-committee includes preparing the programme before the meetings, administration during the meeting, and making the necessary arrangements for publication, if this is desired, after the meeting.

Preparation

The topic or topics for discussion must be determined at least 12 months before the date of the meeting, and potential participants must be notified at that time. This is part of the organisation of the whole meeting, not of the scientific programme. If there is a central theme, and the scientific programme is essentially a symposium, the scope and structure must be decided at this time, and speakers and their subjects selected. The invitation to take part should indicate the intended role of the contributor in the symposium, the duration of his talk, and the subjects covered by the speakers on either side of him. In this way, trespass, duplication, and omission are minimised. Written acceptance of the invitation to speak is essential, and its receipt must be acknowledged by the convener of the scientific committee. If translation has been arranged, you should ask invited contributors to send their full typescript to you at least one week before the meeting to allow translators the opportunity of familiarising themselves with the style, content, and terminology.

The programme of most scientific meetings allows considerable time for papers submitted by contributors on subjects of their own choosing, but usually allied to the main theme. One of the first tasks of a programme subcommittee is to send out an announcement that short papers (generally last 10 minutes) will be included in the programme, and to invite members to submit or sponsor the submission of summaries. If there are to be poster or film and video sessions this should be notified at the same time with the request that intending exhibitors should indicate the size and length of the film or tape and the type of tape. You should prepare a timetable for dealing with the summaries including the following:

(1) The last date on which a summary will be accepted for consideration. To some extent this depends on the size and duration of the meeting, but there are other considerations which are dealt with below and, in general, this date should not be later

than two months before the final day for registration for the meeting.

(2) Decision on how many papers can be accepted. This depends on the time available, and 15 minutes, in practice, should be allowed for a paper of about 10 minutes, so that there is time left for discussion.

(3) Arrangement for the scrutiny and selection of papers. Responsibility for this may be given to a selection committee of three or four people—the smaller the better—who must report to the committee convener within two weeks. This procedure is made easier if summaries are submitted in triplicate on a standard form that is divided into three blocks. The uppermost block is for the title of the paper, the next for the contributors' names and for the place where the work has been done, and the lowest and largest for the summary of the intended contribution, limited to 150 or 200 words. You should already have agreed with your printer the best size for the standard form, and the estimated cost of reproducing the summaries in a booklet which can conveniently be carried at the conference (see figure).

(4) Notification of acceptance or rejection: this must be done at least two weeks before the final day for registration because nowadays university authorities unfortunately may allow expenses to a meeting for junior staff (in particular) only when a paper is being read. In an international meeting where translation is necessary it is also important to be able to give the translators a chance to look at the summaries, as these are the only indication they may receive of the content of short papers.

(5) Printing and distributing programmes. The completed

NAME OF MEETING AND DATES
Title of abstract in capital letters
Author's designation (Prof/Dr/Mr).................................... Initials and name (underlined)...................................... Name of town or city...
The text of the abstract. This should not exceed 250 words. Please use electric typewriter if at all possible

Standard form for summaries

10

programme should be in the hands of all participants 10 days before the meeting, which means being in the post at least four or five days before that.

(6) Reproduction of summaries. The advantage of a standard size and form of summary is that it can be cheaply reproduced by photo-lithography. The disadvantage is that such a book of summaries is usually too big to fit conveniently into a pocket and has to be carried in a folder. Summaries should be distributed with other written matter at the time of registration at the congress. Sending by post beforehand is unnecessarily expensive.

Recording the proceedings

The decision whether a more permanent and fuller record than the summaries is desirable must be made early in the preparations for the meeting. If it is decided to do so, a willing publisher must be sought and a contract entered into with him. The method of recording must also be decided. Broadly speaking there are two ways of doing this. The simpler, but generally less reliable, is to ask contributors to hand in their typescripts to a designated person at a designated place in the meeting hall at the time the paper is given. This designated person would probably be the selected editor of the proceedings, and contributors must understand that he has the usual editor's powers to accept, select, or reject. The second way, which is easier at the time, is to tape-record the proceedings. The advantage of this method is that it also records the discussion. The disadvantage, however, is that the spoken word always has to be extensively edited to make it readable, grammatical, and comprehensible.

If the decision is made to tape-record, it is better to give the job to a commercial firm which will make all the necessary arrangements for recording and for the first transcription. Illustrations normally have to be ruthlessly pruned, for many more are required to point a moral in a talk than to adorn the printed word. If possible, verbal agreement should be reached between editor and contributor at the time of the meeting on the minimum illustrations necessary for clarity.

Organisation during the meeting

Slides—Wrong slides, upside down slides, out of order slides induce more frustration and profanity than any other feature in a meeting and can easily be avoided. One local member should be in charge of slide collection, arrangement, and onward transmission to the projectionist. A slide collection point should be at a prominent place in the foyer and be conspicuously labelled. It is best to have sufficient slide carriages available for each contributor to be given one. *In this he arranges his own slides.* The carriage is then labelled with the contributor's name and the programme number of his paper and is taken by messenger to the projectionist. In this way, all errors and omissions become the responsibility of the contributor himself. Films and videos should be dealt with at the same collection point, labelled, and then passed to the projectionist. Precise instructions are given to the speaker as to the controls of microphone, lights, pointer, and change of slide mechanics.

Chairmen—Chairmen (moderators) of sessions will have been chosen earlier and must have been clearly briefed on their duties, the most important of which is to keep the meeting moving to time. Each chairman must know how to work the platform lights and microphones, and be able to pass the information quickly to speakers. Usually, some means of warning speakers that they are approaching the end of their time is installed. It should be as simple as possible, and preferably noiseless—at least until the final ejection stage.

Discussion—In any large meeting the voices of questioners from the body of the hall will need amplification to be audible to both the speaker and his audience. This may be included in the contract for the halls, but should be checked beforehand, and arrangements made for messengers to carry the portable microphones to where they are required.

III: Registration and its problems

Registration is central to the organisation of any conference and, along with the budget, forms the framework around which the conference is constructed and the timetable devised. It is an exercise in production management, a straight line along which a vast array of details, events, and people have to be programmed. The design of a system of registration is an excellent opportunity for any organising committee to think their project through to the end and, as such, is worth not a little calm and careful thought.

First stages

Ideally, preparation for a large international conference should start two years before the event, and throughout this paper the timing of the various stages of preparation will be given in the number of months away from the opening date.

Organising secretary

A large conference requires an organising secretary who needs a permanent office and staff. On a two-year time scale, the organising secretary should ideally be engaged at 24 months, and certainly by the 18-month mark at the very latest. He is in charge of the conference secretariat, in sole charge of registration, and responsible to the local organising committee chairman and to him alone. The organising secretary services all local organising committee meetings and liaises closely with the chairmen of all subcommittees. He must be kept informed on all aspects of the conference. Policy is decided by the local organising committee and executed by the organising secretary and committee members. Minutes must be kept, listing the duties assigned to the committee members concerned. The organising secretary does not have a vote at committee meetings.

Communication of the conference's requirements to the "outside world" is the most important single function of the organising secretary and, in this respect, we cannot emphasise sufficiently the value of paying a personal visit to everyone whose services will be needed to make the meeting a success. This is especially so with lay people on the committee. In the early days time will be available for this purpose, and it will ease the path towards the final stages when more and more has to be done by telephone. The secretariat will need its own headed paper and telephone number.

The secretarial duties described here assume that the organisation of accommodation—whether in hotels or in university halls of residence—and the allocation of tour tickets are the responsibility of a travel agent, in which case the secretariat need only hold a record of delegates' requirements.

The office

The conference office should be as near as possible to the site of the conference. In the closing few weeks there is an infinite variety of reasons why it is convenient to be near the scene of the final preparations. The office must be large enough to house at least small meetings—say, six people attending—and to store various consignments of conference literature.

The staff

A personal secretary who has knowledge of a foreign language is a boon, especially when multilingual delegates are expected. All outgoing correspondence, however, may safely be conducted in

13

English. At nine months an assistant should be engaged on a morning-only basis to deal with book-keeping and registration records, and at three months a part-time typist should join the ranks of the secretariat. Efficient and interested staff are the greatest asset to this kind of project. It is astonishing how many details of those attending can be absorbed by interested staff and by the time the conference actually takes place you have a hard core of registration personnel with considerable background knowledge.

Accommodation

Having estimated the number of people likely to attend your conference, you must next reserve the accommodation required for the actual meeting in the form of lecture theatres, reception, exhibition halls, temporary offices, and committee rooms. Rooms in hotels and university halls of residence are the remit of the appointed travel agent. Accommodation requirements can often be met by drawing on the resources of your local university, hospital, or municipal offices. Do bear in mind that their facilities are often booked years in advance and that you must act quickly. (See also VIPs and invited speakers.)

Publicity

Progress along the line of conference preparation will be annotated by what you choose to make known of yourselves and at what time. Not uncommonly conference committees produce written information in three stages: the preliminary circular at 18 months; the preliminary programme at 12 months; and the final programme to be collected by delegates on registration. The preliminary circular, in our experience, is unnecessary, since it includes nothing which cannot be contained in a fuller and more satisfying form in the preliminary programme (and it causes unnecessary expense and effort).

Announcements could be placed at 18 months in the relevant professional journals and newsletters, and a mailing list kept at the secretariat of those wanting further details. As a general note on publicity, do not overlook the usual human capacity to misread and misinterpret information, which will be aggravated when not all the recipients speak English as their first language. Instructions must therefore be brief and clear. The problems and expense associated with providing translation facilities are dealt with below and it may well be that, as a committee, you decide against providing this service. None the less, it is worth while to produce information on your social programme at the preliminary programme stage in both French and Spanish.

Distribution

International societies tend to distribute their publications by way of chapter secretaries, to whom circulars and programmes are sent in bulk. Make quite sure that you have the correct name and address of the person concerned and that they send you notification of receipt. Busy professional people have more to do than write letters, so send them a receipt which they or their secretaries may simply sign and return. If these receipts are not forthcoming within three weeks of dispatch, make inquiries. The chapter secretary, if left undisturbed, may very well make no contact with the local organising committee until it is much too late.

Official carrier

An official carrier should be appointed. In return for a free advertisement in conference publications and representation in your registration area, an airline, usually local, will often provide complimentary tickets for use by committee members on conference business and possibly some of your VIPs, as well as free transport of those bulk packages to your various chapter secretaries. Several airlines will approach you in the early stages of setting up your conference. Whichever one you select should state in writing what benefits they offer as official carriers and what they expect in return. Do not forget that these are details which will have to make printing deadlines.

Preliminary programme

The preliminary programme is a major statement of intent: it states who is meeting, when, where, why, and how. The following are details which it must contain:

(a) *Official languages*—These are often English, French, and Spanish. By "official" is meant that a paper may be presented in any of the languages mentioned. Nevertheless, it does not guarantee that simultaneous translation facilities will be provided.

(b) *Scientific programme*—A provisional timetable and list of subjects must be provided along with an application form for contributions. Some important decisions must now be taken—for example,

- what is the deadline for contributions;
- are abstracts of papers to be available during the conference;

15

- what is the time allotted to each speaker;
- if there are both symposia and short paper sessions, do you process the papers differently?

If both symposia and short paper sessions are to be held, then a book of abstracts is prepared of the latter. Preparing the book of abstracts is made much easier by designing an application form to go with a paper, the bottom half of which is divided into three blocks (see figure p 10) giving from the top: the title of the paper, the author's name and address, and a summary not exceeding 250 words. These half papers can be then reproduced by photolithography and bound into pocket-size books.

The vexed question of translation keeps cropping up. In practice the "simultaneous" translators prefer to have a preview of the paper to be presented. It is impossible to receive all the full texts in advance—even for symposia papers only about half of the texts requested are usually received. In these circumstances, translators often have to work from no preparation other than a look at some of the other papers on the same topic. Obviously for short papers the only preparation material available are the relevant abstracts.

You will almost certainly have to limit translation facilities. The choice lies between keeping the translators together in one lecture theatre or in using their services in different locations during plenary sessions or symposia.

At 24 months you must produce a list of VIPs. Registrations should be checked against this list at regular intervals and VIP documentation marked accordingly. First-class accommodation is earmarked for all VIPs and here, a dire word of warning. As a committee, *you* will have made these reservations; as a committee *you* will be liable to pay for it if the accommodation is not claimed. Make quite sure, therefore, that your VIPs know of your arrangements and that they let you know their firm intentions, in writing, by two months at the very latest.

(c) *Categories of membership*—These usually fall into three groups: full members, who may take part in all proceedings of the conference, scientific, technical, and social; associate members, who are introduced by full members, may take part in scientific and technical parts of the conference, and in the social events if space and numbers permit; family members, who accompany full and associate members, may take part in social events only.

(d) *Registration and payment of fees*—In the preliminary programme the cost of the various categories of membership should be stated and a penalty date, six months from the conference, on which fees are increased by an amount agreed by the local organising committee. The necessary registration form, a printed envelope, and instructions that payment should be made by bank transfer to the organising secretary of the conference should also be enclosed.

(e) *Cancellation of registration*—The local organising committee should agree a sliding scale of refund and set the dates on which they apply.

(f) *Reservation of accommodation*—Details of how to apply for accommodation along with a brief description of the various categories available and an approximate price should be stated in full. Make it clear that no reservations of accommodation will be

---

(For office use only)   Reg No

Important. Before completing this form, read carefully the instructions on Page x of the preliminary programme.

Full membership

Surname . . . .   Initials. . . . .

 Title (Prof/Dr/Mr/Mrs/Miss) . . . .   Country . . . .

Mailing Address . . . .

. . . .

Family members

(1) . . . .

(2) . . . .

(3) . . . .

(4) . . . .

Associate members

Surname . . . .   Initials. . . . .

Title . . . .   Country . . . .

Mailing Address . . . .

. . . .

Registration fees

☐ Full members at £A (£A + £B if registering after. . . .) =

☐ Family members at £C . . . . =

☐ Associate members at FD . . . . =

I enclose cheque/bank transfer No . . . . to cover =
 the total cost of my registration fees
and, where applicable, banquet ticket(s)   =
                                                            ——————
                                          Total £
                                                            ——————

Registration form (A4)

Event....................... Date.................. No of tickets
required

Banquet ($£X$ per single ticket).......................................

Date................... Signature......................

Social events form (on reverse side of registration form)

Name ....

Title ....

Mailing Address ....

....

Hotels: Grade A hotel—superior first class
Grade B hotel—first class
Grade C hotel—second class

Number and type of room required

Grade.........Single Room with/without bath

Grade.........Double Room with/without bath

Date of arrival .... Date of departure ....

University halls of residence ....

Number and type of rooms required ....
Single Rooms
Double Rooms

Date of arrival .... Date of departure ....

Deposit—instructions, if any, regarding payment of non-returnable deposit

Accommodation Application Form (A4)

made until the registration fee has been paid. Since accommodation is to be arranged by an official conference travel agent, then it is wise to state that the secretariat cannot undertake to make hotel or student residence reservations. Requests for accommodation will inevitably be made to the secretariat, but these must simply be acknowledged and passed on to the travel agent.

The preliminary programme must also contain the following invaluable information: names and addresses of official conference travel agents, carrier, and bank; officers of the society concerned, including chapter secretaries; local committee members and address of secretariat office; full details of the social programme—however trying it may be to have these particulars arranged one year in advance. Social events include the opening ceremony, trade exhibition, cocktail party receptions, the banquet, and tours of the city and local countryside. (Details of the social programme will be given later.)

Invited speakers

A word of warning on the subject of invited speakers. Not surprisingly, many people will assume that as an invited speaker they need not register in advance or pay a fee, and that their accommodation will automatically be reserved on their behalf. Be quite clear as to the scope of your "invitation" and keep a list of invited speakers. It is necessary even for them to process their registration and to apply for accommodation.

VIPs

We had wanted to say more about the mechanics of registration before mentioning VIPs, but the logical time to bring them in is with this note on invited speakers. VIPs are important, and they do have a right to expect that things will be done for them. Nevertheless, as one or two among perhaps 2000 delegates, their interest is best served if, like everyone else, they too complete the official documentation and go through the one and only mill.

In summary, at 12 months your preliminary programme is dispatched, accompanied by a registration form and application forms for accommodation, social events, and scientific contributions, along with a printed reply envelope to be used for everything except the scientific contribution (which is forwarded to the local chapter secretary). The different forms are printed in different colour for easy identification, and, if nothing else, for an international meeting the social events are described in both French and English. We shall be discussing the mechanics of registration later but in the meantime would like to suggest possible designs for the forms so far mentioned (see figures).

IV: Registration: the mechanics

The first completed application forms and registration fees will start to arrive nine months before the opening date. Do not be disappointed by a slow start. The secretariat must count the heads, collect the fees, and keep the following basic records, all of which stem from the information requested in the documentation sent out with the preliminary programme. It is essential that fees be collected by the local secretariat: do not be tempted by an overseas treasurer to do otherwise.

Basic records in the office

Each individual application to attend the conference is registered in a log book which is written up daily.

Sample page

Reg No	Name	Country	Membership			Fees paid
			Full	Associate	Family	

The log book gives a day-to-day record of the number of delegates attending in any of the various categories. It also gives the name of the delegate and his registration number. This registration number is recorded on the registration form, the accommodation form, the social events application form, and on the acknowledgment card, which are all sent to the delegate.

Registration card

The registration form is awkward to handle compared with a card (see sample) and for this and other reasons the information it

Full/associate member	Reg No
Surname.................... Initial........ Title....	Country
Family members (1) .... (2) .... (3) .... (4) .... Total	
Address for correspondence Conference address in town	
Accommodation requested: Hotel/residence Yes/No No of beds: Arriving: Departing:	

Specimen registration card (actual size 30 cm × 13 cm)

20

carries is immediately transferred to a record card, which is kept in a firm transparent plastic envelope and filed alphabetically according to country. On the reverse of the card should be stated the title of the participant's talk together with the time, date, and place of the meeting. The original registration form now becomes redundant, although we suggest that you do not throw it out.

Social events application forms

Social events applications are also noted in a simple log book. A loose-leaf folder with a section for each event is best. Once again, a day-by-day note is kept of the numbers applying for each event. Once logged, the social events application, along with the requisite tickets (printed in advance), are filled in the same plastic envelope as the delegate's record card.

Accommodation forms

The delegate's registration number is written on to the top right-hand corner of his accommodation form, which is then sent directly to the conference travel agent once the details of the accommodation requested have been noted on the appropriate record card. In due course the travel agent will tell the secretariat where each delegate is staying, and this information will also be noted on the record card.

Let the travel agent bill each delegate direct for his accommodation. Delegates do not always apply in time to get the accommodation of their first choice, and a single account from your agent absolves you from making refunds.

Why not have accommodation forms sent direct to the travel agent?

Largely because you must insert the registration number; also because it is easier for the delegate to post one preprinted envelope to you containing all his particulars; and, lastly, because it enables you to keep your records complete and fully up to date.

Why use registration numbers?

Largely to ease communication between yourself and your travel agent over identifying delegates. Complications may arise over foreign names, and you may have delegates with the same or similar names. Tickets and accommodation must be allotted strictly on a first-come, first-served basis, and numbers are a simple guide to precedence.

Acknowledgment card

Once an application to attend has been logged and placed on a record card *and you have received all fees due,* then an acknowledgment card is sent to the delegate. The delegate must bring this with him as his congress registration card, against which he may complete his registration on site by claiming his congress briefcase. Please note that it is just as important to confirm to a delegate that he has not requested accommodation as it is to confirm that he has.

CONGRESS REGISTRATION CARD

Dear Sir/Madam,

The organising secretary has pleasure in acknowledging receipt of your forms of application and registration fee and notes that you do/do not wish accommodation to be reserved in City X on your behalf.

Name	Initials	Country	Reg No
. . . .	. . . .	. . . .	. . . .

Please present this card at the registration bureau when you arrive in City X.

Secretariat address and tel No

. . . .

Specimen registration/acknowledgment card (postcard size)

The registration area itself should now be considered and also those expressions of your administrative effort, the conference briefcase and final programme. This section will be completed by a brief summary of the procedures outlined.

Briefcases

Stage one with briefcases is to obtain them and, with this in mind, you may safely start looking for a sponsor at 24 months. Briefcases should be robust and will contain the following: final programme; book of scientific abstracts (unless these are to be sold separately); map and general information on city/country; bus map and timetable; advertising material from sponsoring drug companies; and list of participants.

Social events tickets

Remember that tickets for the various social events have over the months been filed along with the individual record cards in plastic envelopes, all stored in alphabetical order, according to country. Ten days before the conference you must produce a list of those attending. Obviously, its preparation should be delayed as long as possible, but ten days from the start should be your absolute limit.

Now is the time to take all the social events tickets and transfer them into envelopes, on which is then written the delegate's name, registration number and country. These envelopes are kept aside in alphabetical order according to country at the appropriate registration desk, so that on presentation by the delegate of his card acknowledging his registration and fee (congress registration card) two things are handed to him. Firstly, the envelope containing his tickets for social events where applicable, plus a stick-on name badge, already completed (which he affixes to his briefcase), and a pin-on identification badge. Secondly, a briefcase containing all the information needed for all full and associate members.

For the staff, therefore, registration is a question of being handed a card, of going through a file of envelopes, and of reaching for a briefcase from a pile of identically filled cases. It should take less than one minute for a delegate to register and be less complicated than buying a railway ticket.

Proof of registration

The delegate's congress registration card is retained by the secretariat and filed along with his record card as proof of registration. This is not as futile as it may seem: delegates frequently wish to check if their friends and colleagues have arrived.

Registration during the congress

For many conferences the registration area has to be improvised, and is normally constructed from a lecture theatre. A typical size for this would be about 60 m × 25 m. There should be space along one side of the registration area for five registration booths, each the length of two average-sized tables. Between these booths you could allocate, say, 56 countries, grouping them loosely according to language and taking care to share the volume of traffic more or less equally. The following are the five registration groups we have found most useful:

(1) Argentina, Brazil, Cuba, Guatemala, Mexico, Portugal, Spain, Uruguay, Venezuela.

23

(2) Belgium, Egypt, France, Iran, Iraq, Italy, Lebanon, Morocco, Saudi Arabia, Tunisia.

(3) Austria, Denmark, DDR, FDR, Finland, Hungary, Netherlands, Norway, Surinam, Sweden, Switzerland.

(4) Australia, Canada, Eire, Ghana, Hong Kong, India, Malaysia, Malta, New Zealand, Nigeria, Rhodesia, South Africa, Togo, USA.

(5) Bulgaria, China, Czechoslovakia, Greece, Israel, Iceland, Japan, Poland, Romania, Turkey, United Kingdom, USSR, Yugoslavia.

Also within the registration area must be the conference bank, post office, travel bureau, information desk, refreshments, and seats and tables for use by delegates. Lastly, the secretariat—complete with extra typing staff for the occasion, Xerox-copying facilities, and all files and records moved specially from your permanent office.

It is vital that no delays occur at registration. Delegates arrive tired and wish to sign on with minimum fuss. To avoid queues at the registration booths, all queries should be referred to the secretariat. Any delegate who is unable to produce a congress registration card should be escorted personally to the secretariat, where the problem should be resolved. The common cause of a problem is usually a lost card (in which case a duplicate may be issued), or perhaps registration fees have been paid late, in which case no card would have been issued. It is not unusual for delegates from Eastern Europe to prefer to pay on arrival.

Queries may also arise over tickets for the various social events and here you reap the benefit of being able to produce, from the same plastic envelope as the record card, the delegate's original ticket application form.

A cashier is essential in the registration area to handle registrations, including day registrations and ticket payments. Life is much simpler if only *one* person handles cash and if they have proper facilities.

Throughout the conference, and especially during peak registration times, members of the local organising committee should be constantly on hand to deal with contingencies and also to introduce themselves to any delegate who looks lost. The impression this gives, and justifiably so, of looking after your delegates, greatly helps the success of the entire project.

V: The final programme

The first important decision regarding the final programme is to be quite sure which committee members are responsible for writing

24

the different sections. Copy must be in press by the two-month mark at the very latest. Ideally, the final programme should be pocket size—15 cm × 25 cm—and should contain information about the outline programme, in both French and English and including both social events and scientific programme; and general information, also in French and English, consisting of:

(1) *Registration and information centre*—Location and times of opening and telephone numbers;

(2) *Congress secretariat*—As above;

(3) *Congress badges*—Explanation of various colours where necessary; note on procedure should they be lost (that is, report to secretariat immediately); and, most important, the request that badges should be worn at all times (see note on security).

(4) *Press office*—Location, telephone, and opening times. The press office should handle all requests for interviews, press conferences, and photographs.

(5) *Trade exhibition*—Location, opening times, plus time of official opening ceremony, and telephone number of trade information desk. A large section of the final programme will, of course, be devoted to the trade exhibition which will give a complete list of all firms attending, their stand numbers, and a profile of their products.

(6) *Travel bureau*—Location, opening times, and telephone.

(7) *Airline office*—As above.

(8) *Banking services*—As above.

(9) *Post office*—A postal and telecommunications service should be provided for delegates from a temporary post office located in X area. The post office will be open from 0900 to 1600 hours, and its telephone number should be given. Outgoing calls may be made from public telephone boxes located at 1, 2, 3, 4 points. The cost of a local call is Xp.

(10) *Refreshments*—State location, opening times, and approximate price. *N.B.* Continental people do not have the same drinking habits as ourselves and providing special lunch bars and beer tents is not a viable proposition. Nevertheless, a bar accommodating about 200 people, open all day and situated in the trade exhibition, should be adequate. Remember that to have your own bar in, for example, university premises does not absolve the committee from responsibility for finding out if special licensing permission must be obtained.

(11) *Medical services*—In cases of emergency the usual facilities would be available, but with a conference held within a university it is a good idea to co-operate with the university medical service, which has regular consulting hours and a resident dental staff. These facilities can be announced in the final programme—but do

25

remember to obtain official blessing from the director of the university medical centre.

(12) *Taxis*—List main taxi firms in the area, giving telephone numbers.

(13) *Self-drive care hire and chauffeur-driven cars*—As above.

(14) *Public bus services*—Details of main city services to and from conference centre.

(15) *Ladies' social programme*—Location plus full details of programme.

(16) *Maps*—Pull-out maps of city centre and conference area. Don't forget to clear copyright where necessary.

(17) *Scientific programme*—Give full details.

(18) *Advertisers*—Advertising is an important source of revenue and should greatly defray the costs of producing the final programme. A committee member should be delegated to sell advertising space, or you may choose to employ the services of an advertising agent. We recommend you do the job yourself. An agent charges commission, often payable also to other subcontracted agents, and he is quite likely to omit many local advertisers whom a committee member could easily contact himself.

Other considerations

Temporary staff

In a large meeting you may need up to 40 temporary staff divided equally between medical students, who should be responsible for slide collection, and arts students, who can act as stewards and interpreters in the registration area. The arts students may be helped by members of the local Women's Royal Volunteer Service, especially for coping with inquiries regarding the city and local districts at the information desk at the time of registration.

The languages that we think it is essential to cover are French, German, Italian, Spanish, and Russian. French is the second language of many delegates from the Middle East and from Eastern Europe, and Spanish speakers are appreciative if, after a journey from South America, they are not obliged to speak English.

It is well worth while to have a safety margin in your staff numbers, as well as having enough people to cover for lunch and coffee breaks. It is essential to have people "on hand" to accompany delegates in special circumstances: for example, to retrieve lost luggage at the railway station or airport, or to accompany someone to the hospital casualty department. To be able to provide a certain amount of handholding makes the important difference between a delegate feeling that he has arrived, and feeling that he has arrived and can now relax.

Official receptions

You will certainly have to arrange at least one official reception: these are some of the considerations in staging an opening ceremony:

(1) *Hall*—Booked from city two years in advance. Ushers and floral decorations may well have to be arranged through separate suppliers.

(2) *Public address system*—A special contractor may have to be engaged, but obviously you cannot discuss these requirements until you have made final plans for placing your platform party.

(3) *Platform party*—Who receives them on arrival at hall? Check the order of precedence for city dignitaries in the line-up. Order of speeches? Drinks before, after, or both.

(4) *Refreshments*—If refreshments are being provided for participants, check on the licensing laws and local rules; for example, no alcohol may be sold in certain halls booked for an opening.

(5) *Orchestra*—Some entertainment before the ceremony is much appreciated. A concert goes down well, but you will have to book the orchestra a year in advance. Do not forget that if your concert is broadcast live or taped for broadcast you may receive a considerable reduction in the usual fee charged by the orchestra.

(6) *Official invitations*—Be quite clear among committee members about who will receive official invitations to attend receptions, and whose task it is to issue these invitations. Also, do not overlook the ease with which it is possible to forget that tickets must be printed for such events, including special tickets for the platform party.

(7) *Programmes*—Don't forget that, once printed, you still have to arrange to have these distributed.

(8) *Flowers*—While on the subject of floral decoration—for the stage at the opening ceremony at least—don't forget that a display of flowers in the registration area or trade exhibition enhances its appearance. All major cities have a parks and gardens department and it is often possible to rent flowers from such bodies.

(9) *Umbrellas*—In the UK, at least, it is wise to have a few large umbrellas available at the entrance to your receptions and people there to carry them.

(10) *Transport*—If special transportation is provided for your delegates, do remember that, in the UK, it is illegal to take payment for a fare or to issue tickets on a hired bus.

(11) *Taxis*—Tell local taxi services about the time and location of your special functions: a queue of taxis by a concert hall exit comes to no harm.

Public relations/press officer

The public relations and press management of any conference are specialist jobs. The university press officer may make you this kind of offer, and, failing this, make quite sure that one person, and one only, is delegated as press officer. The following are intended as guidelines on how to approach the subject, but your first stage should be to form a small public relations committee consisting of, say, four or five members, including representatives from the local press.

(1) *Advance publicity*—At four months from the start of your conference, invitations should be sent by your public relations officer to the national press, TV, BBC radio, and local radio stations, as well as editors of the professional and trade press, inviting them to attend, or, if they wish, make arrangements to cover the conference. The invitation letter should be accompanied by a press release giving the date, location, countries attending, and an outline programme. This information should also go to the Commonwealth Press Union; Press Association; Reuter; Foreign Press Association; and US correspondents in London.

At this stage the press office should compile profiles of newsworthy delegates attending the conference and any items of particular interest in the scientific programme or trade exhibition.

(2) *Advance press conference*—Late during the week before the conference, the main office-bearers should take a press conference attended by visiting journalists, national and local press, TV, BBC and local radio—all invited to attend by the public relations officer. This press conference should cover the whole ground of the following week's proceedings.

(3) *Publicity during the conference*—The press are invited to attend the opening and closing ceremonies, all appropriate scientific sessions, and all social events and receptions. Evening press conferences may be arranged at the end of each working day in the press office, where the chairmen of the various sessions can give an account of the day's proceedings.

(4) *Press office*—A temporary press office should be set up in the conference centre, consisting of the working press office itself and a room suitable for press interviews and sound radio interviews. The office should have available all morning national papers; all current press releases; advance copies of speeches; copies of congress

programmes; general literature on the societies taking part; and refreshments.

The press office should be set up two days before the delegates arrive and should operate until the final press conference has been held.

(5) *Press cards*—These must be available for distribution to press members.

Insurance

The following insurance cover must be taken out by the local organising committee:

(1) *Public and employer's liability*—To cover injury or damage to or caused by committee employees. Inexpensive but essential—indeed, a legal obligation. Cover for £1m can be arranged for a modest premium.

(2) *Abandonment cover*—This figure must equal the irrecoverable expenditure that would be incurred by the committee were the conference to be cancelled at the last minute—due to strikes, fires, epidemics and so on. It must also include such unpaid commitments as perishable stocks laid in by caterers for events that have to be cancelled.

(3) *Briefcases*—These will certainly have to be stored on conference or committee premises, for a few days at least. Make sure you insure against their loss by fire or theft.

(4) *Office contents*—No matter how modest your office, or how many of its contents are borrowed or lent, take out an All Risks policy to cover its contents.

Finally, check that the number of people you intend to accommodate in the various halls and lecture theatres does not contravene local fire regulations. Fire regulations are surprisingly strict and neglecting them could be disastrous.

Security

Unfortunately, it is a fact of life that large gatherings of people (especially in a confined space) attract the criminal element of any community, especially petty thieves. It is therefore essential that a security service be provided. The university security officer can often provide a first-class 24-hour service to cover all conference premises. It is extremely important that delegates should always wear their conference badge. Anyone not wearing a badge should be asked by a security officer to identify himself.

Cleaning

Special cleaning services will have to be arranged for conference premises, including the trade exhibition. Little things like unemptied ashtrays create a bad impression. The best and obvious source of the service is the body from whom you rent the premises.

Temporary telephones

The GPO requires three months' notice to install temporary telephones. Be particularly careful about telephones. *Visit* everyone concerned in providing the service and be on hand to go round the actual location with the installation engineers. Temporary telephone numbers appear in your final programme and they must be correct. It is unbelievably easy to get them wrong. Check each on site. Temporary telephones are necessary but expensive.

Xerox

Your secretariat will require a Xerox photocopier from the word go, and the press office will almost certainly need one during the conference. These can be obtained on a short-term rental and you may be able to obtain more favourable terms by renting through your university or hospital.

Spare typewriter

A remarkable number of delegates will ask for typing facilities, so have a spare typewriter for their use.

Attendance certificates

A popular request, so have them prepared in advance with nothing to complete but the delegate's name.

VI: The social programme

The social programme and the arrangements for entertaining the ladies are subordinate to those of the main meeting, but their importance should not be underestimated. Get the registration right and get the ladies' programme right, and the conference will succeed. From the outset one member of the organising committee should be charged with this as his sole duty, and the committee must decide early on the general form of the entertainment and how much they wish to spend on it. The form is largely determined by the length of the meeting, the custom of previous occasions, and the requirements of protocol. The aim is at entertaining the delegates and their families and, while you should not rely too heavily on inspired improvisation or the natural generosity of the hosts, there is room for imagination and the light touch.

The main events of the social programme normally form a pattern. There is an opening ceremony, receptions, a show or stage performance, a free evening, and a dinner. Closing the conference is usually a modest affair at the end of the business programme. The social programme should not be a major item in the budget. Comparison with previous meetings may help you to decide the level of entertainment. Receptions are usually provided by the civic authorities, university, or local professional bodies. Such potential hosts should be contacted as soon as possible and tentative dates and maximum numbers established. Large formal dinners are much more expensive than they were a few years ago, and individual attitudes to them vary so much, that the dinner, which is usually the last formal social event, is costed separately and paid for by ticket. The main expense of the social programme lies in the opening ceremony. Whatever else fails, the opening ceremony must succeed—so that the available money should be concentrated on this. The possibility of arranging an opera, concert, or theatre performance will, of course, vary from place to place, but in general it is much cheaper to arrange block bookings for scheduled performances than to stage something special. The latter is really possible only if the state or civic authorities will meet the cost.

Some general points

Most of the social programme is in the evening. The timing of events will depend on that of the conference programme but must allow for delegates returning to their hotels to change and dine. A firm decision should be taken about dress at the various functions, and advice about this included in both the preliminary and the final programmes. Availability of transport at night must be borne in mind. If there is an official conference photographer, he should be expected to attend the main evening events, but freelance photographers should be discouraged.

Besides the main events, the committee must think of the facilities available on the conference site. Registration for a large international meeting is a lengthy business, and delegates tend to loiter in the reception area in the hope of meeting friends or making sure that their arrangements are complete. Some lounge accommodation with coffee, and a desk dealing with social events, ease the handling of large numbers. The questions of lunch for delegates, bar facilities, and hospitality rooms are matters for the main committee, and are best considered with the arrangements for the business part of the meeting.

The opening ceremony

The opening ceremony is attended by most of the delegates and their wives. It is an opportunity to invite local dignitaries and those who have helped with the organisation. It is an occasion for the press. The numbers are large, and may demand a hall larger than anything on the conference site. Think big. Spare seats may be filled by enlarging the circle of friends, or by judicious advertisement. If the opening is to be a large affair, it is probably most conveniently held in the evening of the day of registration, before the start of the conference proper. The time will depend on local custom and the hour of dinner in local hotels. Since the ceremony is a form of entertainment, it will last two hours or so, and speeches should be kept short.

Start the evening with a short display or concert lasting 40 minutes. Allow 20 minutes to assemble the platform party and reset the stage. The formal speeches need take no longer than an hour. Their number and order will be decided by the main committee according to protocol. The necessary mood of relaxed anticipation may be prolonged if a wine buffet is in prospect at the end of the evening. Arrangements include signposting the hall, since it may not be on the conference site, arranging flowers in the foyer and on the platform, ensuring that there is adequate transport for delegates to and from the hall, and notifying the police for security and control of traffic. Finally, it is worth considering employing an official master of ceremonies who will be responsible for the platform party and introducing speakers for this occasion.

Receptions and free evening

Receptions and free evenings are no problem, since the hosts will deal with the detailed organisation. The limiting size seems to be about 300 guests, so that it is convenient, at a large conference, to disperse the party among several simultaneous receptions. All that the social committee will have to do is to allocate guests to each, and arrange transport.

It is a great advantage, especially in a large international meeting, to leave at least one night free of formal entertainment. There may well be local delegates who will welcome the chance to repay hospitality and there are often sectional interests within the main conference—regional clubs, class reunions, and the like—which may use the occasion. The latter may be glad of a little space on the printed programme and may ask for a desk in the registration area or a hospitality room.

Hospitality rooms, social club, ladies' club

The question of hospitality rooms arises only at large conferences: they are rooms at or near the registration area where important visitors may be entertained in some comfort, or conference business transacted. The number of hospitality rooms should be kept to a minimum, usually restricting their use to the chairman of the organising committee, the president of the conference, and the press. The rooms should be clearly signposted and should have telephones.

Catering for lunches, a social club, and a ladies' club, are all related and depend on the size of the conference and existing local services. Modern conference centres may take account of all this but, where a purpose-built centre is not used, it is still important to keep all aspects of the meeting as close together as possible. Ideally, the registration area, restaurant, lounge, and bar should be in the same building. Where this isn't possible, the catering should be close to the venue of the meeting. If the conference is being supported by a trade exhibition, the lounge and bar may be sited close to it to attract delegates to the exhibition. When everything can be centred on the registration area there may be no need for a ladies' club but, if one is to be provided, the ladies' committee must decide whether it is to be near the conference site or near the town shopping centre. There are advantages in both.

The ladies' programme

The ladies' programme includes a range of entertainment for the wives of delegates and, indeed, anyone who wants a day off from the meeting. Some of this can be organised professionally: conducted tours of the city or bus tours of the surrounding countryside. But there are questions of home hospitality, coffee parties, and a ladies' club, which must be dealt with by a ladies' committee. At an early stage, it is a good idea to choose a convener of the ladies' committee who can discuss with the organising committee the dates, expected numbers, whether or not a ladies' club will be needed, what should be organised by the committee and what by official travel agents, and what money will be available

33

for a ladies' programme. Once these main lines are clear, she can convene a small committee of ladies which should be responsible for the details and which, much nearer the time, can mobilise such local support as is needed. Arrangements for a ladies' programme have to be rather tentative, because the number of visiting wives remains uncertain until registration, but it is wise to overestimate, especially in calculating numbers for bus tours. Again, during the conference itself, it is better to mobilise too many of the "home team" than too few, as this spreads the load more comfortably.

The ladies' programme should be scheduled during the hours of the main meeting, evening events being poorly attended. Bus tours are always popular. Fashion shows and similar displays are so only if they relate to national dress or customs. Attendance at a conference can be fitted so easily into a package holiday that a delegate may be accompanied by his whole family. It isn't necessary to organise a crèche, but it is worth collecting some information on how to amuse teenagers during the meeting and, indeed, the ladies' committee can help with the production of the printed conference brochure by compiling a list of useful tephone numbers and addresses of shops, taxis, hairdressers, and restaurants (graded according to cost of a meal).

The dinner

The dinner is the most difficult part of the programme to arrange—at least for a large conference. The problems are mostly related to the numbers of guests, and our discussion assumes a meeting of 1000 or more delegates. You can confidently predict that not all will attend the dinner. You may have some information about numbers at previous dinners but, even if only half attend, there will be too many for any hotel not built with an eye to the conference trade. This means using a hall not originally designed for catering and employing a firm of outside caterers. The success of the dinner will depend very largely on the latter, so they must be chosen with care. Use an established firm that is known to be capable of handling the expected numbers. Book them early, settle the venue of the dinner, and get an estimate of the cost per head. Wines form much of the cost, and you can save a lot by buying the wine in bulk as soon as possible to offset inevitable price rises in the year or two before the conference takes place. Any surplus wine can be sold at a profit after the event, so that this is a reasonable speculation.

Common sources of complaint are: too long an interval before dinner is served; slow service letting dinner get cold; not enough wine; inaudible after-dinner speeches. These difficulties arise from handling large numbers of guests. The pre-dinner interval should not be more than 45 minutes, but this time will be needed for the guests to arrive and sort themselves out, and to marshal top-table guests. Generous space should be allowed for foyer and cloakrooms, and plenty of extra cloakroom staff engaged. All wines, including drinks before dinner, should be included in the price of the ticket. It is courteous to meet top-table guests at the foyer and entertain them separately before dinner. It also ensures that they can be seated expeditiously in their proper places.

A big dinner demands a good toastmaster. His first duty will be to announce dinner. For very large numbers an individual seating plan is too laborious, but some sort of order must be imposed. One solution is to give out numbered cards on arrival, each matching one in the dining hall indicating a table or group of tables. The toastmaster can then invite the guests in to dinner by these numbers. Slow service and cold food are due to an over-ambitious menu with too many hot dishes. The first course, paté or hors d'oeuvres and a glass of sherry, can be on the table at the start. A hot soup can follow this, and then a cold main course with hot vegetables if desired, and a sweet and fruit to follow. A menu of this sort simplifies the choice of wine and lets the wine waiters concentrate on seeing that everyone is well served.

A short interval may be necessary between the end of dinner and the speeches. At a very large dinner it is unwise to announce this formally—it may be difficult to persuade the company to resume their seats. Speeches should be brief, clearly announced by the toastmaster, and audible throughout the hall. This means more than usual attention to the position of amplifiers throughout the hall. The toastmaster must be able to obtain silence for the speaker, who, in turn, may reasonably expect to be heard by everyone. The acoustic problems of large halls are often difficult and should not be left until the last minute. It is worth while spending extra money to get an expert to arrange this, rather than an enthusiastic amateur.

One last word. Of all the conference papers, the dinner menu—dogeared, wine-stained, signed illegibly by old friends and new—remains the most durable souvenir. It should start the evening as a pretty thing.

Acknowledgments

The idea for these papers on how to organise an international medical meeting came from the happy association we had with the other members of the organising committee of the Joint Congress of the International Surgical Society and the International Cardiovascular Society held in Edinburgh in 1975 under the stimulating and provocative chairmanship of the late Sir John Bruce. We acknowledge the overall contributions made by Mr George A Hendry, the organising secretary of the Joint Congress; Mr William Reid, treasurer; Mr John McGhee, public relations officer of the City of Edinburgh; Mr Andrew Hay; Mr John Ward; Mr John Cook; and Miss Hannah Harkins.

[1] Capperauld I, Reid W. *Journal of the Royal College of Surgeons of Edinburgh* 1976; **21**: 302.

Chair a conference

RONALD GIBSON

Although much depends on the type of conference—the size, the length, the subject—certain basic principles are common to all.

Firstly, I think it is vital that you have some idea why you have been elected to take the chair. It may be because of age or experience, a reputation for being a good chairman or—and this is well worth remembering—because successive efforts to find some-one else have failed. You might have been low on the list when the conference was first mooted. It is a salutary thought that you have been the first sucker to accept.

Being elected to the chair by the conference itself has its advantages. It is usually the culmination of years of effort on your part or it may be quite unexpected; in either case, you can reckon to have at least a nodding acquaintance with most of the members. The disadvantage is that you may find when you sit in the special chair reserved for the chairman that it isn't a bit like you thought. Suddenly you are alone and isolated from the rest of the conference. Friendly faces previously surrounding you on the floor can now only be seen at a distance. They look nothing like as friendly from your new seat (or is this your imagination?).

Have you, you wonder, a friend in the hall? This may be the first time that you experience that oft to be repeated temptation to cut and run. Resist it. Have a quick look round from your throne as you sit waiting for the clock to tell you it is time to start and make a note of those you see (preferably scattered about the hall) who could form the nucleus of a reliable MI5 for you. This is particularly helpful if the conference lasts more than one day.

However long it lasts, you must expect the sense of isolation to persist; even the buzz of conversation round the bar or in the dining room will suddenly dry up as you arrive to take some much needed refreshment. This may partly be due to respect and (which is much more likely) partly to the traditional but unwritten rule

37

that the chairman must not be party to any opinions they may be expressing or plots they may be hatching.

The lady behind the bar (who has extraordinarily acute hearing), the ushers, or even the hall porter can often, unwittingly, be members of your MI5 ("Good morning, chairman, I hear they've got it in for you today" is well worth the conversation about the weather you shared with him the night before).

In spite of your sense of isolation, however, it is unwise for you not to seem to be mixing with the members during the conference. They like to have a close look at you and to feel that, in spite of the possibly irreparable damage they are doing to your health, you are still one of them and they tend to resent seeing you only at a distance. You cannot afford to be aloof or incommunicado off stage. There is always hanging over you the threat of "no confidence in the chair." You are less likely to be faced with this if you display obvious regret that it is impossible for you to talk individually to each member of the conference (though this is what you would like and may actually feel you've done by the time the conference ends). Do not forget, also, to exhibit commendable humility throughout.

Helpers and others

The first friend you must make is the secretary of the conference: he is steeped in a subject of which you have only superficial knowledge, and without his approval and advice your chairmanship can be constantly at risk. Establish a happy working partnership from your first meeting (which should be well before the conference opens). Ask him to brief you on the subjects to be debated and possible snags. Ensure that he lets you know any particular characteristics of the conference—each usually has its own. Those taking part have personality traits, foibles, paranoias, and motivations that are peculiar to their trade and which it is unwise to disregard. When you know him well enough, gently try to prise from him some of his knowledge of those taking part. This is a delicate subject, but it is always wise to have a list of those capable of making life difficult for you and of others who can be relied on to get you out of trouble: the humorists who may try to take the mick out of the chair (they can turn out to be your best friends), and those who although—in your view—full of sound and fury signifying nothing, must be treated with the greatest respect (if slighted they can be your worst enemies).

Having established a happy working relationship with the secretary (at the same time paying due compliments to his clerk or personal assistant) and given him the tacit assurance of your implicit obedience, next turn your attention to bylaws and standing orders. These are usually inexplicable hell, and it is as well early on to persuade members that you are congenitally incapable of interpreting them. This brings you down to their level without them having to confess their own ignorance. It also has the additional advantage of ensuring that they are on your side when you are challenged by the inevitable member who knows standing orders by heart.

Rigid adherence to standing orders and an inability to stretch them if the conference so wills is unwise. On the other hand, there are two that the chairman must know: the procedure to be adopted on the motions either that "the question be now put," or that the conference should now "pass to the next business." Any hesitation from the chair after these suggestions may lose the confidence of members. It is sometimes possible, indeed desirable, for the chair to anticipate these motions by hinting to a sympathetic member (through a third party) that, by one or other of the available alternatives, a particular debate should be closed—it is as well that some subjects should not reach voting stage and that others should not be overdebated. I believe that at such times it is the chairman's duty and, indeed, his prerogative, to sense the feeling of the conference and help members to disentangle themselves before any permanent damage is done.

Preconference homework having been done, the chairman will take his seat with apprehension, tachycardia, and loss of nerve. These feelings are necessary if the conference is to be successful and they should in no way be distorted by taking alcohol or tranquillisers. Yet, of course, they must be disguised from the members: the chair must present an appearance of calm and fortitude.

The human touch

When opening the conference I suggest that you address the members briefly. You should emphasise that you are, of course, their servant; your object is to develop a happy family atmosphere; you will do your best (you say) to be absolutely impartial and ensure that every speaker gets a full hearing. You add, somewhat regretfully, that they will understand you are merely human and bound to make mistakes, for which you can only throw yourself on their mercy. You then show that you have a sense of humour by including a little throw away quip, and end up by intimating that, despite your acknowledged inadequacies in the chair, you can exhibit a punch like a kangaroo if necessary. This latter comment must, of course, be put over by inference or innuendo and accompanied by a bland and innocent smile, yet there must be no doubt that it is clearly understood.

The conference will then, with luck, proceed peacefully—at any rate for the first hour or two. You must be benign and generous, fixing the members with an occasional smile which they will come to know means you think they are being good and are proud to be their chairman or, on the contrary, that you think they are being very clever but they had better "watch it" before they go too far. This is very different from setting out to control the conference from the word go. I have seen a chairman determinedly stand up to members, in the mistaken belief that, by so doing, he was proving that he is the boss. In fact he was oppressing opinion and antagonising delegates.

With the help of your friend, the secretary, you will soon get to know who is the clown of the conference and who the potential chair destroyer. As I have said, let the first have his way until you sense the conference has had enough. Let the latter have plenty of rein until he thinks he is about to deliver the coup de grâce, and then give a tug calculated to pull the bit through his mouth and halfway down his throat. The timing requires careful calculation because members are watching the battle, they know the rules of the game and will not tolerate any infringement; they don't want it to end before they have seen two or three rounds, yet they will not forgive the chair if its opponent triumphs (nor will the opponent— strangely, he too is aware of his challenge and is prepared to yield to a manifestly better man).

Although a gentle quip from the chair directed toward the speaker is not a bad thing, it must be seen to have a friendly intention. Members don't enjoy the chair being funny or clever at the speaker's expense, but will happily accept a little amicable fun, even though they know there may be a tiny bite attached to it. It is far more likely that members will support the chair (with which they may secretly be in agreement) if they are allowed to set a speaker down themselves; there is nothing to be gained by the chair trying to do this job for them and thus run the risk of switching sympathy over to the speaker.

War and peace

So you will proceed. Peacefully and unobtrusively guiding the debates but never failing to be attentive. Strangely, it may be that you will not take in a word that is being said. This is all right— subconsciously you are keeping one step ahead and you are relying here on the secretary to nudge you if you appear to have missed a vital point. Try to avoid being in communication with an eager member who wants to fire a question at you from over your shoulder—arrange for someone to accept and note such questions and pass them on to you, if he must, between debates.

The more peaceful the proceedings (if you are wise) the more concentrated your attention, for round the corner may be the crisis that besets all conferences at least once. It is what I call the "gadarene swine motion." Often it is initiated by a comparatively unknown, young and enthusiastic member (more dangerously, an attractive woman), speaking to what at first seemed to be an innocent and inoffensive motion. The little fire he or she lights is fanned by successive speakers. Suddenly there is an ominous silence in the hall; the secretary sharpens his pencil (with luck, he warns "this is it"); others on the platform start to fidget; a queue of speakers forms at the microphone; the press is agog, for the conference is about to exhibit its authority over the Establishment, of which you are part. You are on your own and you will never have felt so lonely. Any attempt to limit the length of speeches or the number of speakers, will be noisily resisted. Any show of dissent by the Establishment will be howled down. Members are enjoying themselves—so, at last, is the press. Let it go. Do not entertain suggestions that you pass to the next business or that a vote be now taken. You must play this one and it may take an hour or more. Never lose your grip, yet never be seen to enforce your authority. Hope that the very force of the flames will put the fire out before it is too late. I have never found it productive to try to appeal to the good nature of members—on these occasions they haven't any. Far better to wait for them to play themselves out, then—when the acute phase is over—it may be possible to extricate the conference from the results of its orgy before a vote is taken. More than this you cannot do.

After this, purged and passive, contrite members—suddenly realising what they have done—will be clay in your hands. With pained (but not angry) demeanour you may now lead them through twice or three times more motions than normal. This, together with a soporific after-lunch session, is of immense value to you in speeding through the business of the conference. The suffering you have endured will have been worth while.

Getting through the remaining important items of the agenda now has priority. Before the penitent reaction is over it can be productively used in getting members' permission to pick special items out for debate, putting others aside for discussion later (if there is time). They will almost certainly approve, howling down any dissenters as part of the redemptive process. Although each member will regard his particular motion as of the utmost importance—it is not for you to disabuse him—you must be ruthless in overriding him. Your objective is to finish the day with major decisions having been taken and the raison d'être of the conference substantiated. Once you have done this to your satisfaction you may attend to the rest of the agenda, knowing that even if you don't debate every item, the conference has effectively produced an informed opinion.

At the end, some kind chap (primed to do so by the secretary—if you have not by now offended the latter beyond words) will propose a vote of thanks to the chair. You will be duly applauded by all and sundry—including, you hope, the press—who, although they have appeared to make life hell for you over the past few hours, have really been your good friends and welcome this opportunity to show their devotion.

Now is the time for the double whisky (repeated, if desired) and it is surprising how quickly the pulse rate returns to normal.

I am more than conscious of my failings as a chairman, yet I am fairly certain that they would have been fewer had I been able to stick to the guidelines I have so glibly suggested here.

Chair a committee

A G W WHITFIELD

One out of four telephone calls to a consultant finds him away at, or in, a meeting and incommunicado and three out of four to an administrator meet the same fate.[1] Some of the consultant's meetings are of an important clinical, scientific, or educational nature and some of the administrator's meetings are essential for the smooth working of his hospital, district, or region. However, committees have become an increasing preoccupation of the National Health Service and many of them serve little or no useful purpose. Democracy demands that everybody must be represented and in consequence they grow larger and larger. The majority are held during time in which those attending are highly paid to do other work, considerable travel and subsistence expenses may be involved, and a secretariat is required. Moreover the cost of producing and posting the agenda and other papers is considerable.

No one appears to have published any estimate of the proportion of the health service budget spent on committees; indeed like so many other National Health Service activities it would probably be impossible to do so with any degree of accuracy and even less feasible to assess their cost effectiveness.

Opinions about the Griffiths report are divided but most are hostile. However if the new general managers it proposes can reduce the number of committees and the numbers serving on each committee by one half it would be unlikely to harm the service and it would release a vast amount of money and expert time for the real purpose of the health service—to care for the sick.

A request to be chairman of a committee should not therefore always be regarded as a mark of the high esteem of one's colleagues and eagerly accepted as an appointment of distinction. It may well be that those requesting your services appreciate that the particular committee is a waste of time and that they have been rebuffed by six others already approached. Even committees which only meet quarterly demand considerable time and effort from the chairman

[1] Personal unpublished research.

43

and secretary and before accepting one should ask oneself three questions: Is the committee going to achieve anything? Have you the knowledge and ability to chair it? Could anyone else available do it better? Honest answers will certainly not leave you responsible for many committees.

An acceptance carries with it a heavy commitment if your appointment is to be a success. The time actually spent "in the chair" is small but the necessary reading, discussion, consultation, persuasion, and cultivation of good relationships consume many hours. As chairman you are the most important member of the committee and you have to steer it and carry the other members with you. Your chief lieutenant, on whom you will be heavily dependent, is the committee secretary. If it is a university committee he or she will be a member of the registry, a graduate and someone with considerable personal qualities and experience. The quality of the secretariat provided for college committees is equally high and you will find yourself in safe and protective hands. Naturally it is not possible for the National Health Service always to equal such standards.

It is important that your meetings should always be on the same day at the same hour—if monthly, for instance, on the third Thursday at 4 pm. This allows members to reserve the time long in advance and ensures maximum attendance.

Your secretary should keep an up to date list of the addresses to which members of the committee wish their correspondence to be sent and all letters and papers should invariably go by first class post. Members should receive a letter in good time requesting submission of items for the agenda not later than three and a half weeks before the committee sits. You and your secretary must then prepare the agenda and ensure that it reaches members three weeks in advance so that its contents may be studied and any local opinions and additional information a member requires for the meeting obtained. The order of the items is important. If someone who is not a member of the committee is to attend for a particular item it should be placed first so that he may leave thereafter. The most important items should be taken when attendance is maximal—that is, after the late arrivals and before the early departures. Contentious issues are often best left until the end of the meeting when members will be running out of combative steam and longing for their gin and tonic.

Two or three days before the meeting you should discuss with your secretary how each item on the agenda should be handled. It is also helpful to discuss particularly difficult items informally with any member whose interests are affected or who you know holds strong views.

44

It is essential that you should be there to welcome members when they arrive and that you familiarise yourself with their names and background as early as possible. Tea or coffee should be provided before the meeting which should always begin promptly at the appointed time.

No meeting should last longer than an hour and half, preferably much less. Apart from the expenditure of time members' concentration diminishes and they tend to drift away to other commitments. Long meetings indicate either that you are a poor chairman or that the agenda is too long in which case it is wise to obtain assent for an executive committee comprising yourself, the secretary and at the most two or three others to meet a few days before the main committee and deal with all the minor and uncontentious items.

At the beginning of each meeting you should welcome members, particularly newcomers, and thank them for their attendance. You should endeavour to ensure that everyone present is involved in the discussion at some time so that they may feel that they have made a contribution and if any item has particular relevance to a member's department or special interest he should be invited to speak first and again before the discussion closes. At the end of the meeting you should thank members again for their attendance and provide a stirrup cup before they depart.

The draft minutes should reach members while the proceedings are still fresh in their minds, amendments requested, and thanks for their attendance again tendered.

At the end of each year a brief letter or a Christmas card to members thanking them for their help and interest is greatly appreciated.

If everyone was invariably courteous, considerate, helpful, and unselfish chairing a committee would be a pleasure but they are not and after three or four meetings you will know exactly how each member will react to everything that is discussed and who dislikes who. No one's nature or attitudes will change in middle life and you can only make the best of the members you have by exercising tact, persuasion, and friendship. Your choice of a deputy chairman is important. He will stand in for you if you are ill or abroad and he will be one staunch ally on whom you can always rely. Some members never attend. This may be because they have another more pressing standing commitment at the same time but it usually means that they are not interested and in such circumstances the body they represent should be informed and asked if they wish to make another nomination.

There are less rewarding activities than chairing a committee but not many!

45

Be an examiner

H A F DUDLEY

Examining tends regrettably to be an exercise in back scratching. You invite me and I will invite you. We shall exchange good fellowship and gossip; incidentally there will be the occasional students to assess. In some highly disciplined environments—few unfortunately in the UK—there are set standards, defined curricula, and well established examining techniques. These can make examining not only a pleasure but also a supervisory matter where the need for intervention is reduced to a minimum. As an examiner both in and outside your own school it is essential, during the course of the examination, to observe certain rules. Firstly, do not criticise the organisation, the organisers, or the students. One may be drenched with sweat, unable to think because of background noise, and wholly irritated by the candidates' incomprehension (and I am not only talking about other cultures than my own) but nevertheless try and keep a civil tongue in your head—an exercise I often find difficult. Secondly, do not believe you are important or well known. You may be the author of the last major contribution to the understanding of phytobezoars in Peruvian goats but the hardworking (sic) junior staff member who is organising the examination sees you as just another freeloader whom his professor has recruited and will be happy only when you are gone. Also do not expect to be continuously entertained. The examination is taking place in your host's institution. He still has all the cares and worries which would beset you were it not that you are 100 plus miles from home. Let's hope he has got you organised between himself and his colleagues but if not don't complain.

Thirdly, do submit a written report with a fair apportionment of praise and blame. As a junior many years ago committed to scorn delights and live laborious days in order that the organisation might run like clockwork and my chief (oh scrabjious word) would not be bothered, my major wish was that I would be recognised. Such would include being asked to the examiners' meeting and

46

dinner if that occurred, and both home and visiting examiners should note this. Dissemination of praise to those who work in the stokehold—secretaries, nurses, and porters—can help both you, if you are to return, and your hosts. Remember the Duke of Wellington's remark when asked if he had any regrets about his conduct of affairs—"I did not give enough praise."

Written paper

Essays—Though many studies have shown these to be an inept way of testing candidates, they persist. If invited to submit essay questions it is best to decline or to submit such outrageous examples that they will not be accepted. Only so will you be preserved from the ridicule which you will be able to heap on others when the inconsistencies, double meanings, and frank stupidities in their offerings are discovered. More seriously, keep questions as simple as possible and avoid elaborate "clinicalisation" which is put in merely for window dressing. In both writtens and orals it is important to tailor your questions to examinees' expectations. For example, it is better to avoid a question about malignant transformation in a gastric ulcer in case the local teaching is that this can occur. Try to mark written papers against a model which you have made or which is occasionally given to you.

Multiple choice—Setting questions is an esoteric discipline understood by the few, though practised by the many, which requires long apprenticeship and continued application. It is best done by teams working together. If there is a multiple choice question paper in the examination you should ask if you may read through it and then report on any ambiguities or inadequacies it displays. In spite of fancy statistical analysis it is only by constant independent feedback that MCQs can be refined.

Clinicals and orals

Your self image may be of a person as mild as milk and your view of a viva is that it is an exploration of what the candidate knows in an endeavour to lift him up over the examination hurdle. Rest assured that to the candidate you are inevitably an ogre, the examination a confrontation, and its objective to put him down. If you have been examining for any length of time you can also be certain that distortions and misconceptions about you abound. Usually the stories originated with the reputed behaviour of someone else but they will undoubtedly live on with you. The best you can hope for is that your reputation is of a beast but a just

47

beast. Because of this, though outwardly composed, the candidate must always be assumed to be uneasy and over the top of the arousal efficiency curve—that is, so tense that his performance is prone to fall off when any minute additional stress is applied—much as the performance of a failing heart does under increased load. Three things follow: make an extra effort not to be irascible, difficult, contrary, and ultimately exasperated; allow a warm up period which can be up to 10% of the allotted time; and pose initial questions that are likely to be answered successfully by all candidates.

In the warm up you can (if the examination regulations permit) ask about the candidate's background, present or future intended employment, and prospects. It is then usually easy to make a *gentle* transition to a simple question. It is no use switching from "I knew your father well" to "Just tell me how 2-3 DPG fits into the haemoglobin molecule."

The velvet glove

All questions should start by telling the candidate the particular topic on which he is going to be interrogated: "Let's talk about gas exchange in the lungs," and "Now I am going to ask you about your plans for this patient," are examples of how to orientate the mind. If a glazed expression comes over the candidate's face on hearing this preliminary you must decide quickly whether to repeat the orientation or to try another subject. Repetition usually suffices.

Now that the candidate is orientated and launched on a subject, the next point is to check on one's own standard about his replies. Oral examinations in Britain are nearly always judged on what one might call a "floating standard"—an idea drifting about in the examiner's brain of what this examination requires in knowledge or performance or both. It is unusual for this standard to be well formulated and, though the lack of external reference points does not prevent the system from working reasonably well, it is good to keep some constancy by asking the same or related questions of each batch of candidates. To do so is boring, but may expose, for example, that one or more of your questions is outside the ken of 95% of the examinees. Then it should be eliminated or at least relegated to the last part of an oral that is going well, when it becomes desirable to stretch the candidate's performance in the interests of determining his position relative to others, or because it introduces a glimmer of intellectual light into what tends to be a gloomy task. It is only in the latter stage that one can usually expect a candidate to think as he goes, so questions that require concepts

48

rather than facts are not usually handled well. If you wish to introduce them, an even more careful preliminary build up is necessary. To take a simple example: if I want to persuade a candidate to tell me the difference between the capillary and the cell membrane in the context of water and electrolyte transfer, I start by drawing the total body water diagram and getting the facts about ionic content of extra cellular and intracellular compartments and then—and only then—move on to the question that I want answered. This introduction may give you an idea whether it is even worth going on.

Now some simple "do's" and "dont's." Do interject a word or two of praise or reassurance if a candidate is getting things right, but don't labour the point that he is wrong unless it is necessary to head him off from committing suicide. If possible—and this is difficult—avoid even non verbal signs that there is an error in his reply; instead, shift ground with a positive statement such as "Very well, let's go on to . . ." Resist the temptation to teach when things are going wrong. First of all it will lead to you talking too much (and that, if you are examining in pairs, will irritate your partner); secondly, if the candidate has not taken it in before, he is certainly not going to absorb it in the circumstances of an oral. Don't interrupt a candidate's flow of answers if you can avoid it—he is almost bound to be thinking more slowly than you and it is very easy to get out of synchronisation if he is still perseverating on one question while you are galloping ahead with another. The same thing may happen when you are speaking to him, so it is essential to go slowly and use short well formed sentences which tell him exactly when you have finished and he can start.

Special features of the clinical

What I have written applies to any oral. The clinical examination is a special and complicated case. It is fair to say that no one really knows what is being tested (or, better, what the examiners draw out from it) except that it is something different from written papers or vivas across a table. To recall again the Duke of Wellington, who used to say he carried bits of string inside his head to knot together as occasion demanded, I have no detailed plan for the clinical. I do, however, have an outline: can the candidate show that he has taken a history and elicited the important physical findings? If so, move on; if not, go back and see if he can redeem himself. Can he next identify the problem? Can he suggest appropriate management . . .? And so on. I think this is only fair to the candidates and, furthermore, I believe that it is the examiner's duty to make the method of procedure clear so that the candidate's mind has the chance to run in predestined grooves which are the same as those of his interrogator.

Appearance and deportment

I must express a personal view about both the examiner's and the candidate's appearance in vivas. From the candidate I hope for conformity, cleanliness, tidiness, and eagerness because these are the virtues to which I was taught to aspire. But before consciously or unconsciously deducting marks for absence of these, we should reflect whether we share the same value systems and whether the one we have is right for the age in which we now live. From the examiner I hope for the same virtues. I was sad when I read in a recent GMC report that London examiners still smoke, read *The Times*, yawn, and obviously do not pay attention while a young person is facing one of his biggest hurdles. This is discourteous and unforgiveable even though because of his circumstances the candidate has to forgive rather than complain. Let us hope that such bad practices are never indulged in by those who have read these words.

Take an examination paper

P R FLEMING

Examinations in medicine today include an increasing variety of written papers. The answers required range from lengthy essays to the candidate's marks on specially prepared answer sheets which indicate his responses to multiple choice questions. Firstly, I will consider those questions that require from the candidate an attempt to convey his thoughts to the examiners in continuous prose. Later, I will briefly consider questions requiring very short answers and multiple choice questions.

Essay papers

The traditional essay paper consists of 4–6 questions, on each of which you are expected to write for 30–45 minutes; recently, papers have sometimes included a much larger number of questions, perhaps 15 or 20, to which the answers must be correspondingly shorter. Sometimes these two types of question appear in the same paper and, for this reason (and for many others), it is essential that you read through the instructions printed on the paper so that you are quite clear about what is wanted. Having read the whole paper through and, incidentally, noted whether any, or all, of the questions are compulsory, you should spend a moment or two planning your campaign. If possible, it is clearly desirable to decide at the outset which of several optional questions you will answer but, if the choice is difficult and the minutes are ticking away, it may well be wise to start writing answers to the questions that you have definitely decided to attempt. While you are writing, and however hard you may be concentrating on one question, you may find that ideas and facts about other questions spring to mind, and, if you make a note of them as they arise, you may be able to decide more easily which of the remaining questions to answer.

Whether or not you have to choose which questions to answer, you must be certain, before you start to write, how much time you can afford to spend on each question. This is particularly important if there are as many as 15 or so questions in the paper. If three hours are allowed for such a paper, no more than 12 minutes are available for each question and, of these, two minutes or so will be needed for preliminary thought. Few people can write more than 250–300 words legibly in 10 minutes and you should bear this constraint in mind when attempting such questions. At all costs you must answer the right number of questions as, with most systems of marking, it is difficult, if not impossible, to compensate for the omission of a compulsory question by submitting a brilliant answer of inappropriate length to another.

Something should be said about the composition of the answers themselves. You should study the wording of the question to determine precisely what it is that the examiners require. Unfortunately, this is not always easy but it can usually be assumed, in a traditional "long essay" question, that "Discuss . . ." or "Give an account of . . ." really mean, "Write all you know about . . ." Difficulties may arise, however, when only a brief answer is required. Some examiners are not very expert at setting questions which can, in theory, be answered perfectly in 10 minutes, and you will sometimes have the difficult task of deciding what you (and, you hope, the examiners) regard as essential in such an answer. Nevertheless, most such questions are carefully worded and if you are trying to "Give an account of the clinical manifestations of chronic renal failure" do not waste time on a discussion of the biochemical disorder.

Candidates are usually reminded of the importance of writing good English but I must admit that most examiners, conscious perhaps of their own limitations, pay little attention to this and regard split infinitives with some equanimity. This is not to say, however, that they will not be irritated by gross solecisms in style and spelling, and statements like "the patient should be PR'd to exclude malaena" are unlikely to improve your chances. Some examiners are touchy too about abbreviations, and you should be careful about their use. Such terms as BP, JVP, and MSU are probably acceptable but you should avoid "statements" like "After g-i bleed BV$\downarrow$ → CVP$\downarrow$" as a substitute for "After gastrointestinal haemorrhage, the fall in circulating blood volume is reflected in a low central venous pressure."

Short answers and multiple choice questions

The format of some recently introduced written examinations is such that candidates' answers consist of a few lines, or sometimes a phrase or even a single word. Such examinations include the modified essay questions used by the Royal College of General Practitioners, and the written section of part II of the examination for membership of the Royal Colleges of Physicians. There are therefore few problems in composing the answers, but it is particularly important for you to pay attention to any instructions and to the precise wording of the questions. In the membership examination, for example, the questions are very specific and, if you are asked for two possible explanations of a set of laboratory data there is no point whatever in listing three. Brilliant candidates who may feel constrained by the unreality of this format, should remind themselves that they will have ample opportunity to show their expertise in other parts of the examination.

The charge of unreality has also often been levelled at multiple-choice questions and the point is well taken, particularly by those with considerable experience in constructing them. Nevertheless, the disadvantages of MCQ are outweighed by the precision with which your factual knowledge may be assessed by this technique, and MCQ have certainly come to stay. This being the case, you must learn how best to do yourself justice in such an examination. Reading the questions carefully is important; the standard of these questions has risen considerably in recent years and in well conducted examinations ambiguous questions are rare. It is equally important for you to come to terms with the problem of how much to guess in answering them. If, as is commonly the case, marks are deducted for wrong answers, you may be reluctant to attempt any questions other than those about which you are certain. Such timidity usually means doing yourself less than justice. Wild guessing is pointless, but, just as action in clinical medicine may be necessary without complete information, so candidates should be prepared to "play their hunches" when answering MCQ. On the not unreasonable assumption that hunches are, on balance, more often right than wrong, and, provided that no more marks are deducted for an incorrect answer than are awarded for a correct one, this practice will almost always result in an improvement in your score.

Opinions differ on whether, when answering MCQ, it is better to start by working rapidly through the whole paper, marking (on the question paper itself if this is permitted) the answers to those items about which you are certain or to deal more deliberately with each question in turn, giving each as much time as necessary. On the whole the former method is probably preferable as it "gets marks in the bank" early and allows time for a later review of difficult items. As always, it is important to pace yourself throughout such a paper and, if the answers must be inserted on a special sheet for computer marking, allow yourself enough time at the end of the examination for a careful inspection of this sheet for errors of transcription.

53

Take an examination viva

N K SHINTON

The relative importance of the viva voce section of an examination varies from one examination to another. It may be the final assessment of the candidates and therefore important only to those with borderline results, or it may carry a proportion of marks. In some examinations it may be the method of deciding on distinction or honours. These are matters of immediate concern more to the examiner than to yourself and you should approach all viva voce examinations with the intention of conveying to the examiner the fullest possible extent of your understanding of the subject to be discussed. The candidate's approach may be vital for success, but personalities vary from those who are over confident and aggressive to the shy timid people who find this part of the examination the greatest ordeal. Personality differences cannot be completely overcome, and it is better for you to behave normally and not attempt to act out a part which, to your embarrassment, will probably be detected. A determined effort to be composed is always worth while but, in furtherance of this aim I wouldn't recommend tranquillisers, and hypnotics the night before can leave you overcome by sleep at a critical moment.

The moment of face to face contact between the examiner and yourself is important as first impressions can make a difference. For this reason, if you are neatly dressed you have an advantage over someone who is slovenly or flamboyant. Likewise, your entrance into the room and the way you take the proffered chair may convey an impression of alertness or sloth.

The initial question is usually a general one to give you time to settle down and to allow a rapport to develop. At this stage it is most important for you not to repeat the question while you think out the answer—this is a most irritating habit, and remember that the examiner will be listening to numerous candidates. It is better for you to start talking about the subject and if possible go on until the examiner either indicates that he is satisfied or moves on to

54

another question. In the unfortunate event that you do not understand the question, ask for it to be repeated, or say that you don't understand. If you really don't know anything about the subject then say so, because this fact will eventually be deduced and valuable time will have been lost. You should appreciate that in the time allotted you must get across the maximum extent of your knowledge. Many candidates know the subject but are unable to communicate their knowledge to others.

Testing your ability to communicate is the whole purpose of a viva voce examination. Always avoid vagueness or using words to take up time—no credit will accrue from this. Not infrequently the examiner hands across the table a specimen, photograph, or data for comment. It is a good principle to describe the exhibit and then, if possible, what it represents. At the end of the interview always leave graciously, however disagreeable it may have been, as this leaves a good impression and in borderline circumstances may be influential.

Lastly, a word about distinction vivas. These are a battle of wits and knowledge between an above average examinee and the examiner. The questions are certain to stretch the candidate's knowledge to the utmost but for that reason may be quite enjoyable for both. The process of determining the extent of your knowledge may be long or short, so the length of time taken on the procedure is of little importance.

Take a clinical examination

J F STOKES

So you are taking a clinical examination and are looking for some help to get you over this hurdle—regarded by some as a half hour disaster session, and commonly painted in garish retrospective colours by those who have already tried to jump it. The first thing to do is to ignore the account of the man who said he failed because he missed the diagnosis of pseudopseudohypoparathyroidism in the short cases: it is more likely that he was unable to locate an obviously displaced trachea or found himself at a loss when invited to palpate for enlarged cervical lymph nodes. Clinical examinations are for testing your command of clinical skills, for finding out whether you can *do* things rather than simply remember, talk, and write about them. Don't expect to get by on bookwork; reciting 57 causes of haemolytic anaemia will not excuse your failure to feel an easily palpable spleen.

A live dimension

Though you may possibly have had some experience of showing what you can do with a dogfish, a cockroach, or a dead bacterium, a clinical examination introduces a new dimension, in that you are dealing with a live animal—one of your own species, and one which is quite capable of bringing some personal bias into your encounter. Fear of the unknown patient probably upsets some students as much as fear of the unknown examiner; this anxiety is accentuated by knowing that you will be spending some time alone with a patient, whereas you might normally talk to a *pair* of examiners, one discussing a problem with you, the other listening, which improves your chances of a fair appraisal.

Clearly the first step you must take is to ensure that you get lots of practice in talking to patients and in examining them physically; the more abnormal physical signs you have met before, and the wider the range of personalities you have had to contend with, the

56

better. The latter is particularly important when it comes to taking a history, including a psychiatric history, for which you may need special training.

One of your problems may be the proper organisation of the time available to you, so as to be sure that you don't omit any important inquiry. You will, of course, take the blood pressure and test the urine; some people like to do these things early on so that they don't forget them in the race against the clock.

You must be absolutely confident about your ability to search for the apex beat of the heart, and have a clear plan in your mind as to what you are going to do when you can't find it—percuss the precordium, for instance, remembering that emphysema is commoner than dextrocardia. Be sure that you are comfortable with a knee hammer in your hand and that you appreciate that a niggling henpecking approach to the patellar tendon may be as unlikely to provide a reflex as a smart blow on the anterior tubercle of the tibia. And have some idea of how an ophthalmoscope works. An earlier candidate, taking the view that the examination is competitive, may have left it for you with a $+20$ dioptre lens in position and this will unsight you unless you know how to deal with it; remember that as soon as you lift your head you're going to be asked to describe what you saw, so check the instrument before you start—or carry your own. Though many doctors are arrogant in the way they hope to evaluate the retina in ordinary ward daylight, your examiners will have arranged for a pupil to be dilated if there is likely to be any difficulty (you'd better ask the patient whether he has had drops in his eye—he may have Adie's syndrome).

Don't be too hidebound by your training in a rigid framework of inquiry. Use an auriscope if you suspect the possibility of a cerebral abscess; examine the spine of a patient complaining of backache (this is sometimes overlooked), and the head of a patient with headache (rarely undertaken but capable of yielding impressive dividends in the shape of temporal arteritis or osteitis deformans).

It is more difficult to check on adequate history taking than on physical signs, but examiners recognise the overriding importance of taking a history in clinical practice and you will find that the assessment of this special skill will not be overlooked. Again, you should be flexible; you must be prepared to ask leading questions and to go to the heart of your patient's problem rather than play out time with a routine catechism. Some people may advise you to ask the patient three questions: "What's the matter with you?" "What treatment are you having?" and "What questions are the doctors asking about you?" That such an approach continues to be rewarding is due only to the fact that the examiner is not likely to be with you while you are taking a history (though he will watch you collecting your physical signs). Most examiners are aware of this problem and you will probably do better to take a history in the same way as you would if you were in the outpatient clinic rather than sitting an examination; this will at least protect you from such wrong footing as has occurred when the patient's answer to the first question was "psittacosis," interpreted as "silicosis."

Giving a good impression

As to dress and comportment, "neat but not gaudy" should be your watchword. It is at the clinical bedside test that examiners will try to decide what kind of a person you are and their judgment will have some influence on your final score even if it is not given formal weight. Don't be too upset by this random approach, which is already showing signs of being better organised in some parts of the world; in the meantime there are a number of points to which you can usefully pay some attention.

Wear whatever makes you feel comfortable—some people look excruciatingly uptight in an unaccustomed waistcoat. But don't appear more bedraggled than you can help and be sure that your hands and nails are clean; they will shortly be in contact with another human being who may well be spruced up for the occasion, and it is the least you can do. Give your patient identity; call her "Mrs Robinson" when you are asking her to take off her bra, not "granny," which she may not consider appropriate, nor "my dear," which may well be thought presumptuous on so short an acquaintance. It may be difficult for you, but try to relax; examiners get put out by signs of tension (sweating, overbreathing, and tremor all distract them from their job), and, although you may not find it easy to believe, they really welcome an opportunity for a quiet and uninhibited discussion with you.

If you're a man, you will have to give some thought to what tie you are going to wear; it should depend on how you feel when you get up on The Day—a bow, a recognisable club, or something anonymous—whatever is comfortable—but tuck it in if it is long, as it may exhaust the abdominal reflexes while you are auscultating the left chest. You also have to decide what to do with your hands, which are better out of your pockets.

If you're a woman, you have different problems; heavy rings may be uncomfortable for your patient when you palpate for axillary lymph nodes, long hair may flop over the anterior chest wall, swinging earrings get in the way. Your examiner may be an experienced man who is able to pick up a prophetic whiff of "Je

Reviens," so watch your scent. If you are pregnant and it shows, you should be prepared either for an unnerving display of avuncular concern or for an unusually tough interrogation designed to convince the second examiner that no allowances are being made.

It is no longer so urgent as it used to be to discover the identity of your examiner. Pairs protect, and prophylactic action is taken by examining boards to avoid lethal combinations of examining genes. You will, of course, meet hawks and doves and the occasional peacock, woodpecker, cuckoo, or owl, but don't let this worry you; it will enlarge your experience and you may rest assured that, whatever their avian characteristics, the vast majority of them are trying to find out what you *do* know, not what you don't, recognising that an examination is no more than a milestone in a continuum of medical education.

Let me wish you good luck—you will still need a little bit of this.

Write the MD thesis

CLIFFORD HAWKINS

The degree of Doctor of Medicine (MD or DM) in the United Kingdom is a higher doctorate which is coveted by medical graduates, being equal in status to doctorates in other university faculties; this contrasts with practice in countries elsewhere in Europe and in the USA, where it is solely a qualifying degree like the MB, BS. The award of Master of Surgery (MS or Latin ChM) has the same status and requirement; so much so that this degree was discontinued in the University of Birmingham in 1974, the MD subsequently being awarded to both physicians and surgeons, and this has happened elsewhere. Research interests of both disciplines are similar—a far cry from the days when the candidate for the MS was required to prove his ability at anatomy and the MD degree was awarded by examination, like a bar to the Membership of the Royal College of Physicians examination (MRCP). A doctorate of philosophy (PhD) is also awarded to medical graduates, though it tends to have a lower status, as it is the result of supervised research often obtained at the start of a career. The use of the word philosophy for a science degree is anachronistic: it dates back to the original meaning of philosophy, which covered wisdom and knowledge generally.

History of the thesis

The word thesis is derived from the Greek $\theta\epsilon\sigma\iota\varsigma$. It is defined as "a proposition laid down or stated, especially as a theme to be discussed and proved or to be maintained against attack." In medieval universities students were examined for their doctorate before a congregation of graduates, doctors, and professors of the university and had to engage in a disputation in which the thesis was formally attacked, sustained, and defended. The congregation decided at the end of the day whether the standard of presentation, argument, and defence of the thesis justified his admission as a

60

doctor. Fortunately, any oral examination nowadays is less forbidding and merely complementary to the thesis itself.

The MD thesis is a test more of scientific rather than clinical ability and normally provides some contribution to medical knowledge. The most important quality needed for undertaking it is enthusiasm for original work and for studying a subject in depth. Anyone can present a thesis to their university though obviously time and research facilities are needed, yet some to their great credit obtain it from general practice.[1] It also comes easier to those who have already written articles and received the criticisms of editors.

Anyone intending to do an MD thesis should visit his medical school library and peruse theses already accepted. A room is often devoted to these, all standardised with a similar immaculate binding except for colour. Our university has a different colour for each faculty—for example, the binding is red for medicine and grey for science, and these colours correlate with those on the academic gowns. Some are big and others are slender; one in our library, perhaps a record, weighs 5 kg (10 lb) and consists of three volumes. The smallest is 1 kg (2 lb). Size, however, is no guide to quality; indeed, great length may be due to literary incapacity. A first-class thesis is often small and concise.

Looking at the titles of MD theses will show the wide range of topics, varying from investigation of clinical conditions such as Raynaud's syndrome to experimental work such as the teratogenic action of trypan blue. Other material can be used to support the thesis: audiovisual, tape, gramophone record, a book that the author may have published, or a computer print-out.

Choosing a subject

Professional advice must be sought whether a subject for research is viable; else a candidate may easily set out on a task which is too ambitious. A suitable person may be at hand; otherwise an approach should be made to the head of the appropriate department, such as medicine, surgery, obstetrics, psychiatry, oncology, immunology, geriatrics, pharmacology, social medicine, and so on. This is particularly important for anyone working in isolation from a main university department, as discussion must, from the candidate's interest, take place before work is far advanced, and certainly before the thesis is written. If necessary, the dean of the medical school can be asked to suggest someone. Choice of a subject is easiest when the person is one of a research team with an ongoing programme—provided he does the work himself.

61

The topic must contain sufficient material for a thesis and originality is important, though an excellent piece of work confirming what is known would sometimes be acceptable. There must be a consistent theme. A thesis that is disjointed will be turned down, so that it is no good pinning together work already done on a few vaguely related subjects.

As work progresses it may be given as a communication from time to time at medical meetings. A critical audience may be of great help, especially by making constructive suggestions. Similarly, any opportunity to publish work should be seized. If accepted, an article appearing in a reputable medical journal will act as an incentive. Reprints can be inserted in a special pocket at the end of the thesis, or copied by photostat and made part of the thesis, provided that bridging sections make them part of a logical sequence.

Many theses nowadays require the use of statistics, and expert help should be sought from the start. It is a pity that courses in statistics and methods are not readily available for postgraduate students.

Varying regulations of universities

Administrative details are obtained by writing to the academic registrar of the university and asking for a copy of the regulations concerning the MD degree. These regulations vary: for example, candidates may have to have been qualified for periods from two to five years. Some universities, perhaps parochially, only accept theses from their own graduates, whereas others do not discriminate, provided the person has been working at the university for at least two or three years.

The subject of the thesis may have to be approved beforehand by the board of the faculty of medicine, or the thesis can be presented without any preliminary requirement whatsoever. Sometimes not only the title but the outline of future work has to be sent to and approved by the MD committee, when, after formal acceptance, a period of at least eighteen months must elapse before the candidate can submit the thesis itself. Any plan of proposed work must be thought out carefully; it usually only needs to be brief, perhaps covering two or three pages. This approach is helpful, provided a decision is reached quickly by the committee: otherwise the enthusiasm of the candidate may wane. In some universities an adviser is appointed, unless the candidate himself is a member of the staff, but responsibility for consulting the adviser rests with the candidate.

Signed declarations are sometimes required from the candidate, to certify that the thesis has been composed by himself or that the work is his own, or, if he has been a member of a research group, that he has made a substantial contribution himself, or that he has looked up all references himself. Statements may also have to be made by the head of the department.

Three bound copies are usually required. These have to be sent to the dean and he will arrange for them to be circulated among the appointed assessors. If accepted, the *top* copy must be given to the university library; this dates back to the days before efficient photocopiers, as carbon copies might be illegible. It is customary for the candidate to present one volume to the department in which he works, but he keeps the remaining one himself. There is seldom any limit required to the length of the thesis, but the regulations of one university state that it should not normally exceed 60 000 words, including any appendices and protocols of experiments, and that only in exceptional circumstances should it be bound in more than a single volume.

Theses may be accepted, rejected, or revision suggested; the nature of alterations or additions which will render the work acceptable will be indicated and the time allowed for this is often within one year—though this can be extended at the discretion of the board of the faculty. The degree may be awarded either with or without honours and some universities extend this grading: gold medal, highest honours, honours, commendation, and ordinary degree. Criticism has been levelled against grading, in that it may deter a good candidate who thinks that he must obtain only a top award or that it encourages others to inflate their thesis unnecessarily. The standard required for acceptance of an MD thesis still varies in different universities, though fortunately the days have gone when it could be bought like the MA. Obviously, the higher the standard, the greater is the distinction for the candidate.

Most universities accept a thesis without seeing the candidate, though sometimes an oral examination is requested by assessors so that the candidate can explain certain aspects more fully and results can be questioned. The regulations of some require that every candidate has an oral.

Anatomy of a thesis

The MD thesis is usually written according to a conventional plan, though this can be altered when necessary.

Title—The title should be specific, though comprehensive enough to cover work likely to be done. It should be short, yet sufficiently descriptive, without one unnecessary word. Abbreviations must not be used, for they confuse when translated into foreign languages. Francis[2] emphasises that it must be clear enough to allow instant recognition by anyone in the faculty; discussing theses generally, he writes that some extraordinary confusions have arisen in the University of London and key words have not been clear and so the thesis has appeared in a wrong classification in the library filing system.

Preface—Here the author should state in about 50 words what his object is and the methods he has used, setting out clearly why he undertook the work and explaining what hypothesis he held and wished to test.

Synopsis (summary)—This should describe the contents of the thesis in 200 to 500 words. Most careful attention should be given to it, for the assessor first turns to this to find out what has been done and why. If he cannot understand it, perhaps because of jargon or abbreviations which are not explained when first used, his enthusiasm for reading the thesis will weaken.

Survey of previous work—This should be a study in depth of literature concerning the subject. A critical approach should be taken regarding the reliability of previous work and reasons for any serious differences stated. It is often difficult for a writer to know where to limit his delving into the literature. The reader may be bored by a retrospective ramble giving references of everything, or nearly everything, that has ever been said about the topic, whether or not it is relevant.

Material and methods—This section may occupy several chapters in some theses. New techniques may have been developed and the validity of these will have been tested. The reliability of methods of assessment and the type of statistical analysis will probably be described. The amount of laboratory or other work that the candidate himself has done and how much has been done by other workers should be made obvious.

Results—The reporting of results, which is separate from discussion of their significance, should be given succinctly. The normal range of values should be given in parentheses if the reader is unlikely to know. Often experimental results are best presented as tables or figures, though conclusions based on these must appear in the text. The use of both tables and figures to illustrate results must be avoided. Although only relevant results and successful experiments need be described in detail, unsuccessful experiments and the wrong turnings which are inevitable in all research should be recorded. Comments on the meaning of results should not be mixed with the facts but left to the discussion.

Discussion—Here the results are interpreted, commented upon, and appropriate deductions drawn. This part should be limited to discussion, without recapitulation of results.

64

Conclusions—This leads on naturally from discussion. The candidate assesses his results and relates them to the work of others, which will have been described in the survey of work. He may comment upon the limitations of his research and mention any further work that could be carried out.

References—A record card system for filing references should be used at the start; otherwise much time may be wasted in the final throes when chasing up those mislaid or forgotten. Cards can also be rearranged and put in correct order so that a secretary can type a list directly from them. Nevertheless, the value of a thesis is not measured by the number of references. The worst sin is to include a long list of references which have never been seen or read by the author. Incorrect ones cause an appalling waste of time for others and are likely to be detected by the assessor. No reference should be included unless the author has looked it up himself. Personal communications or references to inaccessible journals should be avoided as far as possible.

References must be listed in a uniform way. The Vancouver style uses the numbering system as here. Each reference is given a number according to the order in which it first appears in the text. The reference in the text is indicated by the number, often set superior to the line. The other main method, the Harvard system, is based on a list of references given in alphabetical order; in the text, the reference is indicated by the name of the author and the date of the work given in parentheses: (Gowers, 1973). The international committee of medical journal editors[3] favoured the Vancouver style. If this is used, it is helpful to put the name and date of the author in brackets in the text at the start and change this to a number in a later edition. Two articles by the same authors in the same year are distinguished by letters (Bloggs and Sissons, 1982a, 1982b). The pagination of papers and chapters in books should always be given. The method of abbreviating journals is important and the titles with their abbreviations are printed annually in the January issue of *Index Medicus* at the start under "Lists of the Journals indexed". If in doubt, spell it out—in full.

Examples of how to refer correctly to a paper, book, or thesis are as follows:

McBurney J J, Meier H, Hoag W G.
Device for milking mice. *J Lab Clin Med* 1964; **64**: 485–7.
Gowers, Sir Ernest (revised by Fraser, Sir Bruce) *The complete plain words*. 2 edn. London: HMSO, 1973.
Mynors J M. *The bowel sounds* Thesis ChM. University of Birmingham, 1963.

Acknowledgments—It is helpful to make a list in order to avoid forgetting anyone. Colleagues should be thanked for any help, advice, and encouragement. It is usual to acknowledge the head of

65

the department and facilities made available and financial help, such as research grants or money donated for drugs or equipment. It is necessary to thank the laboratory or other staff only when they have gone to special trouble and not when they have carried out routine work.

Appendix—This is useful for any descriptions or data which would break the continuity of the text. Tables, case reports, and details of special apparatus can be included.

Illustrations—Charts, tables, and diagrams should be close to the relevant text, and easy to understand. Their sole object is to aid comprehension and not just to duplicate material already in the text.

Presentation and binding

A copy of *Notes on the Presentation and Binding of Theses* issued by the university bindery may usually be obtained from the medical school library. This should be scrutinised carefully and shown to one's secretary. Observation of this advice should result in a typographically well-presented thesis. A badly prepared script may not be accepted.

The length of the average thesis varies from 100 to 300 pages. It is generally not more than 50 mm thick and two volumes are made if there are more than 250 pages. Paper of international standard size A4 ($11\frac{3}{4}$ in × $8\frac{1}{4}$ in; 297 × 210 mm) is used and on one side only. The left-hand margin should be about $1\frac{1}{2}$ in (4 cm) and the right $\frac{1}{2}$ in (1·25 cm); the wide left margin is to allow space for binding the pages. Margins at the top and bottom of the page should be about 1 in (2·5 cm). Double-spacing should be used for the main text, but single spacing for footnotes. If photocopies are used, it is essential to tell the operator that the prints are for binding, so that a binding margin of $1\frac{1}{2}$ in (4 cm) is left and the copy is clear. Sufficient paper should be bought for the whole thesis at the start before typing is begun; very slight variations of size can spoil the appearance of a thesis. Pages must be numbered all the way through. From the start it is a good plan to make three copies of all relevant material such as illustrations. Box files are useful for storing data and other material.

Writing the thesis

No thesis worthy of a Nobel Prize will be rejected, or even sent back for revision, even if the English is appalling. Nevertheless, in all other theses, clear English—which means that ideas are conveyed in the fewest words—is essential. Unfortunately, the pompous polysyllabic word dissertation used in regulations of some universities may easily make the author feel that he needs to do something beyond communicating his facts and ideas. He then works hard to create an impression and so may lapse into a cliché-ridden pomposity and verbosity, frequently a contrast to his conversation. There is then loss of direct and forceful manner of writing which is common to authors as different as P G Wodehouse and Winston Churchill. Various books [4-6] are available to guide the author about this matter if he is not aware of the differential diagnosis of the causes of obscurity in writing. Often he is exhorted to read the best authors to improve his English. I cannot agree. No one can learn to paint by visiting art galleries and looking at pictures. An expert's help is needed to tear the script to pieces and to give practical advice. In some medical departments, manuscripts are submitted to a professional writer before publication. Perhaps one day professional medical editing services will be generally available.

Think before starting to write. Time is wasted when pen is put to paper too soon. All facts and ideas should first be assembled. One method then is to make a book of blank pages by putting typing paper into a spring-clip instant binder. Headings, one to a sheet, are jotted down for different problems and ideas as they arise; the blank sheets are filled in with the facts and any additional information can be added. The pages themselves are altered in a more suitable order as the thesis develops and then the arrangement of chapters emerges. Sometimes a short summary at the end of each chapter helps to crystallise the author's thoughts and guides the reader.

Writing should be postponed until a detailed plan has been made, even as far as outlines of paragraphs and construction of sentences. The first draft may be typed, written (with plenty of space between the lines for corrections), or dictated; sometimes the tape-recorder when used without the script in mind is a menace, for it encourages long-windedness. The word processor saves much time as alterations can so easily be made[7]; otherwise tell the secretary to type the first draft *roughly* as this saves her time. Every unnecessary word should then be excised, meanings clarified, and technical details corrected. Some writers are able to submit a final typescript with little effort. Most will not, and they will be consoled by being in the company of most distinguished writers. For example, Somerset Maugham revised his manuscripts six times; that he had "drastically purged them of words" explains the clarity of his writing as he recalled in his book *The Summing Up*.

67

Assessing a thesis

The number of assessors used for correcting a thesis varies in different universities, sometimes two, or maybe four or five. One or two external assessors are chosen for their expertise on the subject. Each sends his independent report to the medical faculty office. If opinions do not agree, assessors may be asked to consult together to see whether agreement can be reached, and an oral examination to question the candidate on his thesis may be advised. Speed and punctuality in returning the corrected thesis is important, though not always easy to achieve, for undue delay may hold up the candidate's career. Gentle reminders from the administrative staff in the medical school office are useful in hastening this.

An assessor usually has numerous other commitments and his work on the thesis, which is always most time-consuming, often has to be done in the evenings or at weekends. The first impact is its size: an enormous volume or volumes will not endear the author to him. He will probably next read the synopsis and then scan the contents to see whether it makes easy reading. When reading it more carefully he will note whether a critical approach is employed, and will study carefully figures, diagrams, graphs, legends, and statistics. Relevant references will be looked up and a random sample checked for their accuracies.

A major problem in assessing theses may be to find out the attribution of the work. Many projects deal with complicated technical procedures. The author may have done most or all of the work himself, or he may have simply taken routine laboratory results and never even visited the laboratory. The same difficulty arises with previous publications, as nearly all papers have several authors. A note attached to each reference indicating the role of the candidate is most helpful.

Causes of failure or need for revision

A thesis is seldom rejected because the subject is not original enough: more likely it fails because it is disjointed and without a single theme running through it, or if too little work has been done by the author himself.

A number of theses are unsatisfactory and have to be returned to the author for revision. This is a burden to him and can be avoided. Inflation is caused by verbosity, irrelevant text, and wasted space, as when the typist leaves too wide margins and when many unnecessary illustrations are used. Errors that have occurred include misquotations from published work, tables upside down, bad captions to tables, masses of complicated data with virtually no explanation in the text, and statistics which neither support the argument nor make sense; and, most common of all, incorrect references. Also many theses contain literal errors, misspellings, words left out, and so on. Examiners are irritated by such carelessness and become naturally suspicious of work done by a candidate who allows so many errors to go uncorrected in his written thesis. They may wonder whether similar errors have occurred in his scientific work.

Is the MD worthwhile?

Motives for taking up the challenge of obtaining the MD must differ. Some do so because of a sense of personal satisfaction or to pursue a particular interest. Many are encouraged to undertake it because it is a valuable stepping stone in their career. Material may be published while the work is being done or after the thesis has been accepted; work subsequently published should contain some reference to the fact that it has been approved by the university for the award of the MD degree. The thesis itself will be listed in the annual publication *Index to Theses*. The British Library at Boston Spa aims to keep a copy of all doctorates of British universities. Some may have carried out excellent research which, perhaps because of negative findings, is not suitable to appear in current medical journals; this may sometimes be tied together in a thesis, provided that there is a common theme and the material is worth while.

The possession of an MD is also a helpful yardstick for those on appointment committees, for it provides proof of sustained endeavour, of the ability to think critically, and of training in scientific method. Brief details of the work which was awarded the MD should be included in a curriculum vitae. The number of graduates who receive MD degrees varies in different universities. Eight per cent of all MBs qualifying in 1947 had obtained the MD at the end of 1964; figures were as high as 20% for Oxbridge.[8] Nevertheless, high figures sometimes reflect the ease of obtaining the degree in the past rather than the intellectual capacity of the recipients. The recommendation of the Joint Committee on Higher Medical Training for a period of research in the training of specialists may make it easier for doctors to obtain the MD in the future.

The MD is complementary to and in no way a rival to higher specialist examinations and diplomas, which test knowledge and training rather than originality. Few studies have been made of the careers of recipients of the MD degree. Whitfield[9] investigated 75 MDs that had been awarded since this had been changed in

69

Birmingham from an examination to a thesis in 1948. He found that 12 had been elected to chairs, and five to readerships, and that four had become senior lecturers and three lecturers, and 44 of the 75 were consultants or honorary consultants. Ogston,[10] who studied the careers of those who had obtained the MD in the University of Aberdeen between 1931 and 1969, noted that 39.9% were occupying hospital appointments, 25% had achieved academic and research posts; others were in general practice, public health, or administration. These figures support Whitfield's conclusion that the MD is, like a doctorate in science, a recognition of high intellectual capacity and the ability to apply it. It is also a hallmark which sets a seal on a period of successful research.

[1] Williams, W O. *Br J Med Educ*, 1969; **3**: 171–5.

[2] Francis, J R D. *Bull Univ Lond*, 1976; **31**: part 1, p 3–4; part 2, p 3–6.

[3] International Committee of Medical Journal Editors. Uniform requirements of manuscripts submitted to biomedical journals, *Br Med J*, 1982; **284**: 1766–70.

[4] Hawkins, C F. Speaking and writing in medicine. *The art of communication*, Springfield: Thomas, 1967.

[5] Lock, S. *Thorne's better medical writing*, Tonbridge Wells: Pitman Medical, 1977.

[6] Huth, E J. *How to write and publish papers in the medical Sciences*. Philadelphia: ISI Press, 1982.

[7] McDonald, P. Writing a thesis on a word processor. *Br Med J*, 1984; **289**: 242.

[8] Wilson, G M. *Br J Med Educ*, 1966; **1**: 58–61.

[9] Whitfield, A G W. *Br J Med Educ*, 1967; **1**: 359–62.

[10] Ogston, D. *Scott Med J*, 1970; **15**: 297–301.

Give a reference

Not another request for a reference—the second in this mail, and the third so far this week! If you have been irritated by a similar experience, it merely emphasises your need to make an appointment with yourself and take the time necessary to formulate a policy for the future. Having made one, stick to it, unless the need to improve the policy becomes obvious. A request for a reference means that somebody values your opinion, needs your help, and believes you will be willing to give it. Remember that you might not have been in the position to receive such requests if someone had not written a reference to support your successful application many years ago for a much desired post leading to your professional success. He or she was possibly just as busy then as you are now, and probably busier, so be prepared to repay the debt by writing a reference for someone else.

Look again at the three requests now awaiting reply. The one for S O Slow need not detain you long. You have had no communication from him since he left your department five years ago, not even a note to bring you up to date on his recent exploits, a curriculum vitae, or a letter to say he was giving your name as a referee. His record may have improved, but five years ago it was not outstanding, and all you remember is that you were no happier to see him leave your team than he obviously was to go. These recollections would not increase his chance of success, so a card from your secretary regretting that you had no information on which to support his application and wishing him well, would be a kind way of dealing with this request, and might help him to behave more courteously in the future.

The second request is on behalf of U Twerp. You remember him well for a variety of reasons, not least of which is that he was one of the only twins to work in your team. They did not hold posts simultaneously. The elder brother had shown more initiative than his younger companion, even while still in utero, by arriving in this

71

world 35 minutes before him. Thereafter, he slowly but progressively outpaced him. When the elder Twerp applied successfully three years ago for a senior registrar position in a busy provincial teaching hospital, you gave him such a splendid reference that he was actually congratulated at the selection interview on the support he had received from you. A somewhat sarcastic personal letter you received a few months later from the head of his new department contained the following passage, which temporarily distressed you:

"I have just read once again the reference you sent in support of the application made by Mr B Twerp for a senior registrar post in this hospital. You are obviously not interested in ornithology, and cannot distinguish a swan from a goose. What you said about his clinical ability was reasonably accurate, but he is so allergic to work that you must have seen him in a remission period, if in fact you saw him at all! I thought it only fair that as his former referee you should know that his appointment to this hospital has been a disaster."

Fortunately for both you and him, the younger Twerp does not request a reference for that hospital, but, of course, the challenger of your refereeing ability could be on the selection committee none the less. Perhaps in the interests of you both, you should decline the request to give a reference for the second Twerp. Now you have had a moment to think about him, perhaps you would agree that he could not be recommended without some reservation. Following the example of some of the consultants and registrars with whom he has been associated, he has become a rather militant member of the "work to rule" brigade. If your reference mentions this he is unlikely to be appointed, and if it fails to do so you may receive another derogatory letter when the truth is apparent soon after his appointment to a new position. Yes, on second thoughts it would be better not to send a reference for Mr Twerp.

The third and last request is from Miss A Winner, who is just completing her appointment as registrar in your hospital, and wishes your support for her application to secure a senior registrar post in a much larger department, before going overseas to spend her professional life working in the Punjab in a Christian Medical College with heavy clinical and teaching responsibilities. Your only hesitation in writing this reference will centre on the mingled feelings with which it will be written. You are anxious to help a most worthy younger colleague, while at the same time you are sad at the thought of losing her from your department. Your expression of these sentiments will provide more help to the selection committee than would an unnecessary paraphrase of the candidate's curriculum vitae, to which they are more accustomed. They already know the appointments she has held but not the use she has made of them. Your comments on this can be vital. Her dedication and motivation, capacity for work, compassion and genuine interest in her patients, her technical skills, the lucidity and quality of her concise, carefully dated and signed records in beautiful, legible handwriting, and the respect and affection in which she is held by students and professional and ancillary staff, are the hallmarks of the excellent doctor you will be unhappy to lose and they should be looking for. Say so in your reference, and remember to comment on her good health record. If she is not shortlisted for interview, the district health authority should review the membership of the selection committee and look for some modern Oslers to replace them.

After these reflections your policy for handling requests for references should be taking shape. To write one should be a pleasure and not an ordeal if you are selective, honest, accurate, relevant, and concise. The result should encourage the selection committee to short list the candidate for interview. If this happens you will both be on trial, with the candidate's performance and your credibility at stake.

Conduct a selection interview

GEORGE DICK

It is unfortunate that the medical profession, apart from those involved in the Services, has not devoted more time and research to methods of assessing the personality of medical personnel which might have provided a background for career guidance and appointments and could save hours of time of interview panels; industry is a long way ahead in this field.[1] Be that as it may, the inteview panel will remain the main selection device for many years to come.

Interviewing panels

In attending interviewing panels, I often used to recall a reproduction in one of my school books of one of Yeame's paintings—"And when last did you see your father." This picture shows a party of Roundheads interviewing a little boy while his family wait in fear in case the boy's answers to questions lead to disaster.

While an interview, properly carried out, should be a two way exchange it must always be remembered that everything is heavily weighted against the candidate.

The numbers on the panel, including a committee officer, should not be more than six or seven, and must include the candidates' future immediate "boss." The sensible candidate will have met him before the interview and will have visited the place of work. He will also have discussed the post with other members of staff, including personnel officers or administrators, one or other of whom may be on the panel (indeed they may have made an order of preference before the formal panel interview).

Preliminaries

An interview is a two way process; the candidate and the interviewers must be properly prepared. The former has probably

74

been coached for the part, but the latter may require some training[2] in gathering information and in assessing the suitability of candidates for the particular jobs. Before the interview a careful study should be made of the job description, the curriculum vitae and the application forms; this will weed out some of the applicants and confirm that the candidate is suitable for interview, for it will be possible to make inferences of his ability—for example, from his attainments and of his stability and health from observing his periods of unemployment, etc.

Before the candidate is interviewed the chairman should ensure that all members of the panel have been introduced to each other; the panel must agree on the procedures to be adopted, and in my experience each member of the panel should concentrate his questions on one particular facet of the job or of the candidate. The chairman should indicate for how long he expects each candidate to be interviewed and that the business should be finished at a given time. In my experience it is fairest to withhold discussions about the suitability of any candidate until all have been interviewed. If the usual procedure is not known, arrangements should be made with administrative officers to ensure that the candidates arrive at intervals of about 30 minutes and not all at once and that waiting time is occupied by paying the travelling expenses of the candidates, checking addresses, and providing any additional information such as the names of the members of the interviewing panel.

Process

Members of the panel should sit round a table and each should be identifiable to the candidate by a nameplate in large letters which also indicates whom they represent (nothing elaborate is required—a folded piece of stiff paper and a felt pen). Unless they are well known to him, the chairman should be given a seating list of the panel; if it is not provided he should make his own.

How to start

If it is not practicable for the chairman of the panel to welcome the candidate with a handshake he should at least stand up when the candidate is brought in and invite him to be seated. If I am chairing the panel, I then usually say to the candidate "You probably know a number of the members of this committee, but just let me introduce them to you" and proceed to do so. With a committee interviewing many applicants it is then advisable to identify each candidate: "You are Dr X and you are applying for the post of registrar in psychiatry at Y Hospital." (This may prevent upset, embarrassment and a waste of time when the panel discover that they are interviewing the wrong man for the wrong job!)

Next you must let the candidate play himself in; he should be asked some general questions of an open type such as: "*How* did you travel?" "*When* did you leave home?" "*Where* exactly is your hospital?" so that he can hear the sound of his own voice. The chairman should then explain how he intends to conduct the interview and should then ask the candidate if he wishes to add anything to the information which he has provided on his application form—for example, the candidate may have completed an examination for a college diploma since applying for the post. All this leads to the candidate developing confidence to play his part in the act. He should be asked if he has read the job description and has any comments on it and if it seems to suit his requirements. The chairman should then invite each member of the panel to interview the candidate.

Questions

It is important that each member of the panel establishes rapport with the candidate. This will be determined by the type of questions which are asked. An interview can be a very trying experience and nothing is gained by starting an interview with a question such as "What is the biggest mistake you've ever made, Mr A?" (A favourite stock opening question by a particular surgeon.) Stress questions can come later if they seem to be indicated. To begin with the members of the panel must attempt to get the best out of all candidates and not just from a favourite.

The questions asked to begin with should be open questions which usually begin with the "Six honest serving men. . . . Their names are *What* and *Why* and *When* and *How* and *Where* and *Who*." The questions asked should be aimed at finding out attitudes, experience, and suitability and should not take the form of a tutorial or a viva for a higher degree, which the candidate may have just recently passed: this of course does not mean that clinical questions or recent work should not be discussed in moderation.

Direct questions have their place in establishing or verifying faults on the application form, but it is always more pleasant to try to phrase these questions in an indirect way, not "You returned to Ruritania for one year in 1980?" but, "What did you do when you visited Ruritania in 1980?" "How long were you in Ruritania?" If the members of the panel fail to fill in lacunae it is important that the chairman should pick up inconsistencies at the end of the discussions. Except to protect the candidate, he and other members of the panel should, however, refrain from interrupting the candidate's discussion with other members of the panel: their turns will come.

I have already indicated that stress questions play little part in a selection interview unless clearly to identify glaring deficiencies which have been concealed by the applicant. Personal questions on religion, politics, and privilege should be excluded and only those family questions which may relate to housing, schooling, etc should be considered. However, with proper preparation the candidate should have obtained domestic information from the personnel department of the hospital or institute before the interview. "What if," or fantasy questions, can often provide useful data on attitudes. We all have favourite questions of this type. I like to ask candidates where they see themselves in 5 or 10 years time and also what research they would do if they suddenly received a large grant and technician help: "What is the one thing you would like to discover?"

Evaluating

In deciding the suitability of a particular candidate I have always tried to have numerical scales. The items which I used to score varied according to the post, but could include personality (empathy), qualifications, service experience, research work, specialist and administrative ability—these headings may be subdivided as necessary and each scored 0–4 or 5. In the case of general practitioners the items to be scored should also include premises, organisation, attachments, partners' share of work load, etc.

It is always worth making a note of the applicant's appearance even if it is just to help to remember him when attempting to decide the most suitable candidate at the end of a long series of interviews.

Experienced interviewers appreciate how easy it is to make erroneous judgements on appearances: while a patient might fail to relate to a surgeon with blue jeans, it could be ideal dress for a doctor in establishing confidence with a patient with a pychiatric illness.

In the past few years a considerable amount of work has been done by industrial and occupational psychologists and by others on interviewing techniques. Perhaps some doctors (although it should be basic to their training) have missed out (as I had) on much information which is available on this subject. Not only does the interviewer need a framework which can be based on something like Professor Rodger's seven point plan—attainments, general

77

intelligence, special aptitudes, interests, disposition, and circum-stances[3] but we should be trying to make decisions not just based on impressions. I do not agree with Professor Eysenck's views on the validity of the interview as a selection device—"You may as well toss a coin".[4]

After the questions have gone round the table the candidate should be asked if there are any questions which he would like to ask the chairman or other members of the panel. Following any further discussion the applicant may be asked if he would accept the post if it were offered to him and either asked to wait to be told the decision of the panel or that he will receive it by letter in a couple of days. The interview procedure is then repeated with the other candidates but often changing the order in which the members of the panel interview the next candidate.

Decision making

After all the candidates have been seen, I prefer that their suitability should be discussed by the panel before looking at their references. The chairman should ask the members of the panel if they consider that any of the candidates should be eliminated without further discussion. He should then invite a senior and experienced member of the panel to sum up the qualities of the remaining eligible candidates: after that the other members of the panel are invited to contribute their opinions (the individual with the highest score may not be the winner because of heavily weighted contraindications).

The chairman should then ask for the references to be read and read between the lines (I was told that all references given by Einstein were the same and said "A B is in the running for a Nobel Prize"). Panel members should also try to give the references a numerical weighting. Some referees may have a biased opinion about a particular candidate. (If a damaging reference is going to be given then I think it is better not to give one at all. Such references can follow people around; it should be a rule that photostat copies of references are not made. Following the "leaking" of what I thought was an honest reference which I gave many years ago, I now try to *read* the references to individuals who have asked me to write one for them.)

After the references have been read the chairman should invite one of the senior members of the panel to place the candidates in order of merit. This is then discussed in turn by each member of the panel and, if agreed, the job is nearly finished. If there is no clear agreement, there will have to be further discussion. It is best to try to obtain unanimous agreement and it is better to make no

78

appointment than to choose someone who does not really fulfil the requirements of the job.

If one of the candidates is recommended for appointment he is often invited back to the committee room after all the applicants have been seen: he is congratulated by the chairman and a starting date, etc, may be briefly discussed, but all such details should be left to the officers of the committee to arrange outside the committee room.

I prefer that the candidates do not wait to be told the decision. If the candidate who is offered the job then refuses how does the second choice feel about taking a post at which he is considered second best? I think a letter should be sent immediately to the selected candidate and once he has accepted the job (by return of post or by telephone) the unsuccessful candidates should then be informed.

Minutes and manners

A minute of the meeting should be kept with the names of the members of the panel and with a short report on each of the candidates based on the framework of the interview. Only by starting to keep such data will we ever progress towards the validation of the panel selection technique. Furthermore, if efforts are made towards a numerical expression of the job profile, comparison can be made with the aptitude and suitability of the applicants,[5] for most validation studies have shown that mistakes in selection are made more regularly than people like to admit. A panel interview like an examination is an act—"a two-man drama" the candidate is trying to put up the best possible appearance and so should each member of the panel. Candidates may be coached for meeting panels of examiners—most of us know quite a number of tricks; some interviewers also require to be coached.

Personal interviews

All I wish to say about personal interviews for counselling, for posts, or for problems, is that a dated record (including the year) should be kept. This should include not only notes taken at the time of the discussion, but also conclusions and recommendations. I kept a separate confidential note book for this purpose.

Epilogue

And what about the follow up? Sometimes one of the candidates with the highest "score" fails to get the job because he or she is too

79

specialised or because of lack of experience in some special requirement or for some other correctable contraindication. In these and other special cases, the regional postgraduate dean or one of the consultant members of the panel should informally let the unsuccessful candidate know that, although first choice of the committee, he or she was not appointed for some particular reason and help should be given to remedy the defect and encouragement to apply for a similar post: counselling is no part of an interview panel's remit but it is an important epilogue.

[1] Occupational Personality Questionaires (to be published) (Saville and Holdsworth Ltd) see Selective Tests Purpose-made Personality Questionaire. *Personnel Management*, 1984; Feb: 47.
[2] Bayne, R. and Fletcher, C. Selecting the selectors. *Personnel Management*, 1983; June: 42–4.
[3] Highaim, M. *The ABC of interviewing*, London: Institute of Personnel Management, 1979.
[4] Palmer, R. A sharper focus for the panel interview. *Personnel Management*, 1983; May: 34–7.
[5] Bolton, M. Interviewing for selection decisions. Personnel Library, NFER—Nelson Pub. 10 Daxville House, Windsor, Berks, 1983.

Assess a job

A J ASBURY

Sooner or later the doctor has to apply for jobs, and this chapter deals with the problem of assessing a new post. The information is intended mainly as a prompt so that applicants will remember to ask all the relevant questions. Obviously some matters will be of greater interest to consultants than more junior staff and vice versa.

The campaign

Unless times are particularly hard one should consider a new post as the next step in a well organised plan to get you to your career goal, and therefore each move should have objectives which you must fulfil. This may be, for example, additional training in a medical specialty, or a lighter job to give you time to read for an exam, or possibly a jumping off post where you can acquire useful referees to get your consultant post. Time spent discussing your career plan with a local faculty adviser will be well repaid. Careful study of the manpower market as described in the DHSS document *Health Trends* will also be useful.

Forewarned is forearmed

The bush telegraph which permeates the medical world will usually give warning that an interesting post is likely to be available, and this is the time to start your preparation.

Use the library to find out about the staff and the hospital itself. Are there any special facilities, "big names," suitable referees etc? The *Medical Directory* can give a good clue as to the ages of staff and allow an estimate of when people will retire. If your plan requires a certain person to be your future referee, then estimate his age to make sure that he will still be around when you need him for the next step.

You should also begin to assemble your curriculum vitae, but don't get it finally typed yet. Other chapters in this book give useful advice on this.

First contacts

You should already be looking out for the advertisement, and as soon as it appears ring up and get the details and an application form. Also request general details of the hospital, and ask for a specimen contract. Any reluctance to produce a specimen contract should be treated with suspicion since there are several hospitals who produce idiosyncratic contracts.

Make arrangements to visit the department, and emphasise the fact that you would like to talk to several people, and have a look round. Try to avoid Friday visits as people tend to be away. You will have to make specific appointments to see, for example, the chairman of the division, the local service organiser, etc. The more senior the post the more people you must meet.

Once the details arrive compare them with your career plan. If they fit in, then complete the application form and your curriculum vitae in the style requested. Don't forget to ask your referees for their permission before quoting their names and do supply them with copies of your CV. Also check the specimen contract, and if you have any doubts contact your local BMA office for advice. Depending on how the closing date for applications fits in with your visit, you may be able to avoid posting your application and be able to deliver it by hand.

The list

Start your preparation for your visit by assembling a list of questions to ask, remembering that some things are better asked of an administrator and some of medical staff. Use the items below as a prompt and modify and augment them according to your own convictions and requirements.

Finance: incoming

What is the salary? When would you get your next increment? Are there other sources of income—for example, cremation fees, visits, etc? Will you get your moving expenses and other financial assistance which doctors normally expect? Are there possibilities for private practice?

Finance: expenses

Will you be able to afford the sort of accommodation that you require? Remember to consider the house prices and rates. What is the likely cost of travel to and from work? Are you expected to pay for parking at the hospital? Will there be school fees and other additional expenses related to children's education?

When checking on one's likely financial situation ensure that not only are you entitled to a certain benefit but that it will actually be given.

The job itself

Does the post give you what you need for your career plan? Does the post carry the required accreditation with the relevant supervisory bodies?

Ask particularly about specialty rotations as these can be very deceptive. For example you may discover that certain parts of the rotation will be available only when you have completed all the less attractive parts. You may find rotations where access to certain parts is restricted to local trainees. It is important to discover who really controls the rotation, and what sort of say you have in your assignment.

Inquire carefully about the exact nature of the work. Remember "extensive paediatric experience" can mean dealing with lots of minor hernias in children farmed out by the teaching hospital.

Check carefully on the on-call system. Find out how flexible it is, you might need extra flexibility to attend a professional course. Who does the rotas? What happens in the case of sickness? Do you have to live in when on-call, and if so is any payment for accommodation required? Is the accommodation reasonable?

Further education in post

Will you be allowed to attend a relevant professional course in the neighbourhood, and will you get your expenses? Will this still hold if there are staffing problems? Will you be allowed to attend the relevant conferences, and will your expenses be paid?

Research

What facilities are there for research? Is research actually encouraged or is it considered to be an annoying necessity? Will you be given time to do a project related to your work? Is there somebody to type the resulting manuscript? Are there facilities to get bits of equipment made? Is there enough space?

The future of the post

If this move is to be your last before retirement it is important to consider the implications of current and future Government policy for the post—for example, the Short report. Could the on-call arrangements change so that a consultant is first in line?

The visit itself

Remember that though this is not "the" interview, it is time for a mutual appraisal, and it is important that you present yourself well. It is definitely the time to dig out the "funeral and wedding suit" and give it a trial run before the interview. In the atmosphere of the informal visit you may well have a better chance to make a good impression than at a formal interview. Use it well!

Take a copy of the job application and your CV with you, and if you have written papers, take some reprints; this is often a good "conversation starter." Don't forget your "prompt list."

Take some food with you; many hosts offer coffee but most forget that you have been on a train for four hours before you arrive, and make no allowance for hypoglycaemia.

Make sure that you arrive on time in spite of industrial action on the railways, buses, and so on. Remember that it can take ages to find a department in a big hospital; it may even be in an annexe two bus rides away. Make sure you have time to freshen up before the appointment.

Arrive at the appointed place at least five minutes early, and introduce yourself to the secretary. When you are introduced to your host make sure that he has got your full name correct; you don't want any good impressions to be wasted on another candidate with a similar name. For the same reason try to be sensibly memorable, so that your host remembers you at the interview—for example, "the girl who paddled a canoe in the Olympic Games."

When you talk to your host remember that you are a guest, and try not to "interview" him, but ensure you cover all points of importance. Few people will object if you say "do you mind if I make some notes while we talk." Don't forget to thank him, he may have cancelled his game of golf to see you.

When you have an opportunity to talk to other members of staff, try to establish whether they are happy in their work, since this might indicate your future state. Beware of the person who is very discouraging. He might be doing you a favour; alternatively his brother might be applying for the same post, or he might just be one of those people who does not fit in anywhere. It is often

84

valuable to cross check the meaning of the job description with staff actually in post.

If you are reasonably pleased by what you see and are confident that you want the post then place your application in the hands of the administration department. At least with the receipt in your hand you can be sure that it has arrived safely. If you are not sure then send the application as appropriate by post, preferably by recorded delivery.

As you leave the area it is worth getting a local newspaper to get an indication of the local house market, and the names of estate agents. Once you have got the names of estate agents from a newspaper you can always phone for details from home. It is often worth buying a local map, particularly if you are reasonably confident of a move.

As soon as you can, probably in the train, complete your notes on the visit. There may be several weeks between your visit and the interview and inevitably some details will be forgotten, so keep your thoughts and impressions safe on paper. Even if you do not apply for the post, your notes may be valuable later when a similar post comes up.

Back to the referees

After your visit it might be helpful to discuss the post personally with your referees. They may well appreciate information which would help them to write the most fitting reference.

Finally . . .

As medical unemployment grows, competition for posts increases, and the well prepared will have a definite advantage, particularly if they can turn the informal visit to their advantage.

Prepare a curriculum vitae

EOIN O'BRIEN

"Name, address. Excuse the fantasy.
Photo of the woman I was at twenty.
Marital status: no second finds me the same.
Virgin, mistress, single and married—
Must I conform to a particular brand?"
PATRICIA MCCARTHY, Curriculum Vitae

I owe a debt of gratitude to an attractive blonde secretary who once graced the offices of a Midland dean of postgraduate studies. Having kindly typed my application for a registrar post, she remarked in her characteristically forthright way—"This could belong to any old fool. Let me rewrite it for you." When she presented me with her interpretation of my medical prowess, it took me some time to accept the metamorphosis. I had been given an astute practical lesson. It is, indeed, a sad reflection on our medical schools that we should emerge brimful of matters medical after six years, but utterly untutored in the art of acquiring an appointment—a tedious business that may occupy much of our time. Thanks to my mentor I am now able to see things from the other side of the fence, and I realise that I was not the only one unable to prepare a curriculum vitae. The standard of curricula vitae submitted for posts at all levels is often abysmally low. At times one is left wondering if the applicant has received any schooling in the rudiments of English spelling and writing.

General layout

There are many ways of planning a curriculum vitae, and the method proposed here (see below) is a personal choice. There are other methods and styles every bit as acceptable. The style chosen, however, should have order and be neatly laid out. It is important to comply fully with the instructions for applicants; if 20 copies of a curriculum vitae are requested, 20 copies must be submitted,

86

however unreasonable this may seem to the applicant. Likewise, if a photograph is requested, one must be supplied. Applications must reach the right person before the closing date. Allow plenty of time for delays in postage and in the hospital distribution of mail.

Many hospital authorities make it difficult for the applicant by providing a totally inadequate application form. The best way of dealing with this problem is to submit your own curriculum vitae, and to complete the form only to draw attention to the corresponding page of the curriculum vitae. Sometimes the application form seeks information that would not normally be included in the curriculum vitae—for example, previous salaries. The advice of your consultant or a colleague may be invaluable.

Suggested layout for curriculum vitae

General and personal

Name: ....

Address: ....

Nationality: .... *Date of birth:* .... *Family:*....

Interests: ....

General education: ....

Undergraduate career

....

(*a*) *Medical school:* ....

    Date of entry: ....

    Date of graduation: ....

(*b*) *Teaching hospitals:* ....

(*c*) *Distinctions:* ....

Postgraduate career

Qualifications:

Previous appointments:

Present appointment(s):

Career plans:

Publications:

Addresses:

Learned societies:

Referees:

87

Typing/printing

With the advent of the word processor the task of keeping a curriculum vitae up to date has been made much easier. Once a curriculum vitae is on a disc (always retain two copies) it can be updated with ease for each job application without the trouble and expense of retyping the entire document. For doctors well advanced in their careers the task of committing what may be a substantial tome to disc may appear daunting, but as curricula vitae are demanded not only when a change of appointment is contemplated, but also for grant applications, pharmaceutical trials, and membership application of learned societies, the effort will be well rewarded. Moreover, if one's career is productive it is surprising how easily publications and achievements are omitted unless they are entered regularly, say on an annual basis.

In the first edition of this book doctors applying for senior posts were advised to have their curricula vitae printed. This expensive exercise is now no longer necessary. With skilful use of the word processor a tastefully designed and error free curriculum vitae can be produced inexpensively. A daisywheel or equivalent printer should be used to provide a high quality typeface. The curriculum vitae can then be photocopied on top quality paper, and for senior appointments the additional small cost of professional photocopying and binding in hard papers is worth while.

Details

Interests—This refers to general interests. These might be considered under the headings "cultural, sporting, or recreational." Any distinctions in these general pursuits should be briefly mentioned—a cap in rugby, for example, or a place in the college or university debating society.

General education—Schools attended, examinations taken with results, and distinctions should be briefly listed.

Undergraduate education—This should include date of entry to and graduation from medical school, and all honours and distinctions should be listed. It is surprising how often applicants fail to mention an honours in examination, or a placing in a prize examination. If there has been a genuine reason for failing or postponing an examination, particularly if this results in a delay in graduation, this should be briefly indicated—for example, family illness preventing the taking of finals on schedule. If, on the other hand, there are no mitigating circumstances the dates should merely be stated.

Qualifications—List full titles of degrees and fellowships with dates of award.

Senior house officer to

Professor Oblong,   July 1972—June 1973
Department of Medicine,   (12 months)
University of Maydell and
St Magdall's Hospital,
London.

Professor Oblong was professor of medicine at the University of
Maydell. His special interest was gastroenterology. There were
40 general medical beds and 10 gastroenterological beds. The
hospital was on-take one night in four and I was on call one
night in three. I gained experience in acute medical emergencies
including acute coronary care. I assisted at Professor Oblong's
outpatients twice weekly at which 2000 general medical problems
and 2000 gastroenterological problems were seen annually. I was
trained in endoscopic procedures, liver and intestinal biopsy
techniques, and was competent to perform these procedures
without supervision at the end of my appointment.

St Magdall's is a teaching hospital at which 300 medical students
attend. I gave two senior and one junior tutorial to the students
each week and participated in the professorial department's
clinical teaching sessions, which were held three times weekly,
and also at the weekly CPC. I gave six lectures to nurses each
term and took part in the general practitioner postgraduate
luncheon meetings.

I participated in a trial of a new H_2 antagonist, and assisted at
experiments to determine the efficacy of the drug on canine
gastric secretion. As a result of this work there has been one
publication (see publications), and another is being prepared for
submission.

Previous appointments—These should be in chronological order.
It is best to put designation of the post on the left hand side of the
page, the tenure on the right, and a summary of experience beneath
this, using the unwritten headings "service commitment," "teaching," "research," or "administration" as appropriate to maintain
order and to help you to remember past experience.

Present appointment(s)—The layout is similar to the above.
There may be more than one post—if one was registrar in medicine
and tutor to the medical school, each post would be dealt with
separately. In the example shown, the greater emphasis is on a
service commitment. This would not be the case in an application

89

for a research or tutor's post. For more senior posts administrative experience would become relevant.

Publications—Accuracy is important. Interviewers often check publications—more to familiarise themselves with the standard and content of the work than to verify its existence—and, understandably, a poor view will be taken if the publication cannot be located. Full details of publications—the full title, each author, and the journal (or book), the year, volume, and page numbers (according to the Vancouver style)—should be given. An asterisk may be used after (or before) those publications in which your contribution was a major one, and this may be indicated in brackets at the head of the list.

When publications become more plentiful in the course of time, they should be classified as original papers, abstracts, editorials or leaders, book chapters, reviews, letters (only those that contribute to the literature should be cited), and miscellaneous writings.

Learned societies and committee membership—These should include not only learned medical societies but also cultural bodies that may indicate your involvement in the arts or community affairs. However, if you do list the Forty Foot Bathers Association be prepared to expound on the qualities that justify its inclusion as a learned society. Committee membership serves as an indication of your administrative experience, and if you have served as chairman or secretary this should be stated.

Scientific communications—These should be listed only if you have personally delivered the address. Presumably, if you are a participant in work being presented by another member of the department, your contribution will be acknowledged when the address is published as an abstract or scientific paper. The full title of the address, and the name, date, and venue of the symposium or meeting should be given. Poster displays at major scientific meetings are often published in abstract form and would therefore appear under the list of publications, but it is reasonable to indicate experience in this form of presentation by putting the title of the poster with the place and date of the meeting followed by a note indicating the appropriate publication. (Avoid the temptation to fatten your curriculum vitae by making one piece of work appear at first glance as a number of separate contributions. It is, however, quite reasonable to indicate the progress of a piece of research through different phases of development, for example, from presentation at a local meeting to presentation, perhaps as a poster, at an international scientific meeting, to publication as an abstract and finally to full publication as a scientific paper.)

Referees—Referees are essential to all applications for jobs and careful thought should be given to their choice. Obviously, it is important to choose a referee who will speak well of one. Some doctors have a habit of asking for an open reference on completion of a post but this will usually be refused, and if given is not worth the paper it is written on. Permission to use a referee's name should always be sought in writing *before* submitting the application. Occasionally time does not permit this and a telephone call may have to suffice, but this should be the exception to the rule. Always give the referee details of when you worked for him—he may have forgotten all about you! It is a good policy to let each referee have a copy of your curriculum vitae. Also give details of the post for which you are applying, and the likely date of interview (if he is away, his secretary will let you or the interview board know this). An interview board is not impressed if the named referees have not sent references, and usually the fault rests with the applicant, who has not allowed sufficient time for the preparation, typing, and delivery of the reference. Allow at least three weeks between the time of posting a letter of request to your referee and the interview.

Dear . . .
   I wish to submit my application for the post of Senior Registrar at St Margaret's Hospital. I enclose a copy of my curriculum vitae and the names of two referees.
Yours sincerely,

Covering letter—A handwritten letter should accompany all applications.

Writing a curriculum vitae is a difficult but important task. Do not leave it until the last minute when that friendly secretary you had in mind is the popular choice of your colleagues who are also seeking new jobs. A slovenly curriculum vitae may be judged as the product of a disorderly individual and an indication of performance. If such is not the case the error for the misconception is entirely one's own; if, on the other hand, the temperament of the applicant is indeed a trifle lacking in discipline and order, the composition of a curriculum vitae may serve as the first exercise in correcting that defect.

Be interviewed

JAMES OWEN DRIFE

Taboo for many years, interviews are coming out of the closet—at least as a subject for medical articles. Several doctors have recently offered hints [1-7] for both candidates and interviewers in articles that are well worth a detour to your local library—though thanks to our professional conservatism the advice of past decades remains equally valuable.[8-9] You may feel that cold-blooded preparation for such a personal affair is unBritish, or that it may even deaden the spontaneity of your performance. However, an interview, like parturition, can be more painful when you don't know what to expect, and you should be better able to relax and do yourself justice if you know the format and some of pitfalls. Don't be diffident about asking advice from senior colleagues, but be prepared for bland or enigmatic replies as they may be reluctant to dogmatise in this delicate area. Ignore the anecdotes of your contemporaries: with interviews as with postoperative complications, those with most experience are not necessarily best qualified to give advice.

I have now moved to the other side of the table, but even now that it is a chore rather than an ordeal, the interview is still taken seriously and is never the mere formality it sometimes seems in retrospect. Some candidates appear well armed with qualifications and experience but do not fit into a committee's plans for a post. A "sitting" candidate may have an appreciable advantage if he is well liked, but even the most popular of "home" candidates courts disaster if he ignores the rules of the game. Don't be overawed if you find yourself competing with a "home" candidate: if you are *on* the shortlist, assume the job is there for the taking.

A heterogeneous committee

Appointment committees for hospital jobs vary in size, tending to become larger along the journey from student's bench to regius

92

chair. "Guidelines" exist about their composition for lower-grade posts, and there are statutory regulations at consultant level, but in general the committee will include representatives from each hospital concerned, a member from another district, a lay person, and (for higher appointments) a contingent from the local university and someone from the appropriate royal college (or, in Scotland, from the National Panel of Specialists). The meeting is arranged by harassed administrators and the chairman may not know who his fellow selectors are until a day or two beforehand. As well as representing different—even conflicting—interests, the members often vary greatly in seniority. How can the candidate impress such a heterogeneous group?

A few generalisations will apply. You should dress to reassure, not to provoke. By most people's standards doctors are quiet and conservative, and interviewees should dress soberly without gratuitous flamboyance such as suede shoes and bow ties. However, within the narrow limits of medical acceptability it is a good idea to stand out a little, and a useful compromise for men is the shameless wearing of a club tie—ideally, a university blue—as a conversation piece. This is recommended only if the candidate is entitled to wear it. If you are a woman you will have worked out, during your years of undergraduate exams, the mixture of femininity and professionalism that suits you best.

When you enter the room you should, in the words of one surgeon, "Go in looking as if you're going to enjoy it." This does not mean entering like a soprano taking an encore at Covent Garden, but it does mean looking a little more relaxed and assertive than you would for a viva exam. Don't worry if you blush or tremble perceptibly: interviewers are familiar with the effects of the autonomic nervous system, and allow for them. You should sit in a businesslike attitude, and your manner should be friendly and alert with just a whiff of authority—similar, perhaps, to the impression you think you give when talking to patients. Look first at the chairman of the committee, who will try (not always successfully) to put you at ease.

Questions and answers

Answering the questions themselves is simple—in theory. All you have to do is project the right mixture of confidence (without bumptiousness), charm (without sycophancy), intelligence (without being overpowering), good humour (without hilarity), enthusiasm (without recklessness), honesty (tempered at all times with tact), and maturity (without senescence). Answers should be neither brusque nor loquacious. Balance is all important. Gen-

93

eralisations like these trip too easily off the tongue, like speeches at a prizegiving, and it might be more helpful to give examples of specific questions.

Candidates for junior posts will be asked in which direction they see their careers developing and why. Candidates for lecturer posts will be asked if they want to become professors. Women candidates will be asked quite pointedly about the role of women in medicine. Candidates who have switched specialties will be asked about the role of orthopaedics in psychiatry, or whatever the relevant change was. You will be asked what attracted you to the job, and about any unusual features (such as unexplained gaps) in your curriculum vitae. Most committees will ask about research that the candidate has done or intends to do. Candidates for more senior jobs will be asked about recent government reports relevant to their specialty. These are bread and butter questions and the way to get them wrong is to look as if you are working them out from basic principles without having thought about them before.

Interviewers are interested in what makes a candidate tick. It is not unknown for interviewees to be asked if they smoke or whether or not they go to church. Surprising importance may be attached to hobbies and interests outside medicine, but be careful to avoid giving the impression that these interfere with your work. The committee wants you to reveal something of your personality, so take the opportunity to talk frankly about your virtues.

There may be trickier questions intended to impress the rest of the committee with the questioner's sharpness as well as test the candidate. In general the interviewers want to help you relax, but if people on the short list seem identical in competence and pleasantness it is legitimate to try and grade them according to their response to demanding questions. "What is your weakness?" "What is wrong with your present job?" "If you were given *unlimited* funds for any kind of research, what would your priorities be?" There are no right answers to the heavier questions, but the candidate who makes tart or glib reply is unlikely to stimulate a spontaneous round of applause. Keep cool by reminding yourself that only the better candidates are asked the most difficult questions, and if you are struggling remember that other members of the committee will be sympathising as you try to cope with their difficult colleague.

Putting yourself across

In times of difficulty platitudes often reveal their deep meaning, and I have to include advice that may seem hackneyed but bears repeating. Be courteous. Be honest: it is futile to try to put over an insincere impression. Memorise what you have written in your curriculum vitae. Look as if you are interested in that particular job, and not as if you are there simply because you want promotion. It goes without saying that you will have visited the department before the interview—such visits are *not* regarded as "canvassing"—and if you meet a member of the committee at your preliminary visit, the impression you create then may be as important as that at the formal interview. At the end of the interview you will be asked if you have any questions: don't ask about pay or holidays. It is acceptable, and indeed desirable, to have no questions.

The kind of advice given here has been criticised[10] for encouraging "yes men." Committees say they like candidates to state their opinions and defend them, but in fact they do not like such defences to be too successful. I have assumed that you are going to your interview because you want the job, and that it is not a kamikaze attempt to change the interviewers' attitudes to life. Your aim should be to convince the committee that you would be a delightful colleague: if you realise you would find them intolerable to work with, you need not accept the job if they offer it to you. The interview is not in fact a battle for survival but a courtship ritual: for the unsuccessful suitors there will be other, often more attractive, opportunities, and for the lucky winner the hard work is just beginning.

[1] Rhodes, P. Interviews: sell yourself. *Br Med J*, 1983, **286**, 706–7.
[2] Rhodes, P. Interviews: what happens. *Br Med J*, 1983, **286**, 784–5.
[3] Oldroyd, J. Finding a practice. II: The interview. *Br Med J*, 1981, **282**, 371–2.
[4] Cohen, B J. How to interview candidates. *Br Med J*, 1983, **286**, 1867–8.
[5] Sturzaker, H G. Survival of the fittest? *Br Med J*, 1979, **ii**, 374–5.
[6] Zorab, J S M. Applying for an appointment in anaesthesia. *Anaesthesia*, 1980, **35**, 601–6.
[7] Gilston, A. Applying for an appointment in anaesthesia. *Anaesthesia*, 1980, **35**, 1217–18.
[8] Proteus. How to apply for medical posts. *Lancet*, 1949, **i**, 34–6.
[9] Stewart, R H M. On the art of being interviewed. *Lancet*, 1971, **i**, 127–9.
[10] Baumslag, N. The pursuit of preferment. *Lancet*, 1971, **i**, 596–7.

Work abroad

ANNE SAVAGE

In times past the decision to work in what was then generally known as "the mission field" required long thought, involving, as it did, a lifetime's service, discomfort, isolation and not a little danger. On the other hand, continuous interesting work was assured. The situation is now reversed, so that easy travel and communications, short contracts, safety, and reasonable comfort must be set against the formidable problems of re-establishment.

That being so your first objective, if you contemplate spending even a short time abroad, must be to secure, so far as possible, your return. Much will depend on your status when you go, but for those already established on the specialist ladder seek out a sympathetic consultant, and discuss your plans: research the possibilities of a future job. The subject of proleptic appointments—that is, those made a year or more in advance—is under discussion, and a few exist. They certainly bring a sense of security to the troubled mind, but be warned of two possible problems. You may find it difficult, because a replacement is lacking, to return on the appointed date, and you may change your mind. If your ambitions are towards general practice then the time spent overseas may count as part of your general professional training, but there are no rules, so approach your postgraduate dean. Keep in touch while you are away and keep a log of "interesting cases." It will provide fascinating reading for your old age, and may prove useful before that as evidence of experience and ability. Do not neglect research. The Third World is so full of unexplained problems that a reasonable project could easily be devised and carried through, even in the absence of sophisticated equipment.

When to go is most often a matter of circumstance, but those in a position to choose might consider the following points. It is easier to study and pass examinations if you continue in an unbroken succession of posts; you will get more out of your time spent abroad if you are already some way up the professional ladder. This applies especially to surgeons and obstetricians; you may be able to incorporate your overseas appointment into your training programme. As mentioned before, this mostly applies to GPs, but a few specialist "accredited" posts exist. Inquire at the appropriate royal college if in doubt; if, as is possible, experience of other disciplines leads to a wavering in your dedication, a move is more easily made at an early stage; if children are involved their education must be considered. Up to seven the local school will serve; after that the cultural differences become sharper, and, apart from a few good international schools, the choice lies between boarding school and home tuition.

Where to go? No problem as to country because of the global shortage of doctors. Avoid South America unless you are proficient in Spanish or Portuguese. Parts of Africa are francophone, otherwise the "lingua franca" is English. Religion rarely causes difficulties, statements such as "strong Christian commitment required" being self-explanatory, but many mission and ex-mission hospitals, even when staffed by religious orders accept recruits of all faiths, or none. Race may occasionally deter; Indians are not accepted in some African countries, and some African nationals may not travel to South Africa. Consider carefully the type of hospital, often designated by the number of doctors on the establishment, (not necessarily the number in post at any one time) and unless you are very self confident, and a handy general surgeon, avoid the one doctor ones. Promises of back up by a nearby centre are worthless if the only road has been washed away by rain.

The choice made, set about getting your papers. In almost all cases a work permit and registration with the medical council are necessary. Forms can be voluminous and forbidding. They are devised by the public service departments with the object of sifting out the dross, of which a fair bit floats round the Third World. Do the best you can; details of your kindergarten successes are not necessary if you have completed university education, but do read the small print, and remember a commissioner for oaths is not necessarily a notary public, and only the latter may certify some photocopies. At the same time write direct to the medical superintendant, or a senior doctor. Sending agencies cannot be expected to be fully up to date, and departments of health are often very vague, and sometimes positively misleading, about conditions at the periphery. It is as well, before the spouse and children step wearily into their new home, to make sure it has some furniture and means of cooking. In addition to the basic questions—housing, shops, schools, and recreational facilities—make a list of the smaller things that might cause problems: voltage, refrigeration,

97

radio reception, availability of any regular medicines, and contraceptives. Do not forget a car. Public transport is mostly overcrowded and unreliable and taxis are scarce and expensive and rarely used by the cognoscanti. A second hand vehicle may be available, but if not, with an eye to spares, find out which make is most favoured locally.

Between decision and departure gather as much information as you can. Medical superintendants desperate for staff can paint a rosy picture and make extravagant promises. Forewarned is forearmed, not necessarily frightened off. Contact with somebody recently returned is invaluable, and students on electives, in particular, can be the source of unbiased and uninhibited comment. Start list making. Little things mean a lot when you are miles from the nearest shop, and even further from "civilisation." Old *BMJs* may serve as toilet paper; nothing substitutes for soap.

It is easier to settle if you know something about the country, its history and people. Hunt the libraries and consider attending a course. Some professional preparation is advisable, though it is comforting to realise that, even in the tropics, most of the patients will be suffering from "European" conditions. Books and audiovisual aids are helpful for those unable to attend a formal course, and informal education may be arranged in the host country. Fortify yourself against cultural deprivation by taking or arranging for the supply of cassettes and any hobby materials. Most importantly, if travelling as a pair, one of whom is not medically qualified, consider the role of the partner. It is essential that he or she be willingly involved and an active participant. Failure to work through this problem has lead to contracts, sometimes the marital one, being prematurely terminated. As with so many aspects of Third World living, the problem is more psychological than real, for in places where talent is so short anyone healthy, flexible, and willing will soon be pressed into service.

Flexibility is, indeed, the most important quality to take with you. Couple it with a degree of circumspection particularly with regard to politics. Although it is true that the major problems of the world will only be solved by political action this is not true at the local level, where partisanship may divide, alienate, and ultimately destroy all you have attempted. You may find the local people watchful and uncommunicative at first, so learn enough of the language and customs for basic courtesy. Failure to greet formally or shake hands may be greatly, if silently, resented. The reward for this slight trouble will be genuine friendship. In the hospital honesty is the only policy. If you don't know something, say so. Medical cowboys, like medical tourists, are distrusted and resented, and, except in the few establishments still boasting long serving medical superintendants, information is rarely "de haut en bas," more an exchange between peers.

Most of the anxieties that afflict intending travellers disappear on arrival. Perhaps a few can be dispelled here. With the exception of areas of war or anarchy you will probably be safer than in the UK, and there, as here, the main danger is from traffic accidents. Given adequate prophylaxis against the obvious hazards—malaria and so on—the incidence of disease is probably much the same, gastrointestinal replacing respiratory incidents in the rich tapestry of daily life. Do not fear being stranded; help and hospitality are universally to be found. New techniques are easier to learn when the mystique which surrounds so much British apprenticeship is dispelled. If, after sufficient time for mutual adjustment, incompatibilities persist, transfer to another hospital can usually be arranged.

Finally, at times of doubt and uncertainty, cling to two undoubted facts. Far more doctors working overseas stay on after the end of their contract than return prematurely, and many who originally came as students or immediately after registration later return as mature doctors. In fact your main problem may be, in more than one sense, "adapting back."

Books

ABC of Healthy Travel, London: BMA Publications, 1983.
Brits Abroad, London: Express Newspapers, 1980.
The Daily Telegraph guide to working abroad.
Preservation of personal health, LSHTM.
The care of babies & young children in the tropics.
Travelling with young children, Nat Ass for Maternal & Child Health.
Paediatric priorities in the developing world.
Werner, D. *Where there is no doctor*, London: Tropical Child Health Unit, 1980.

Publications

The Guardian Weekly.
The Expatriate. Obtainable from The Editor, Rectory Rd, Great Waldingfield, Sudbury, Suffolk, CO10.

Courses

Institute of Child Health. Several short courses of which the best is probably the Paediatric priorities one. But heavily booked up to two years ahead. £80 for one week.

Centre for International Briefing. Farnham Castle. £495 for one week.

VMM Courses three times a year. Last 5/52. Residential. Christian commitment expected. Book 2/12 ahead. £350.

Oxfam, three evening meetings; good programme. £8.

Women's Corona Society. ODA. One day courses. I think will accept men. Individual briefing. £20.

Schools of Hygiene and Tropical Medicine, both in London and Liverpool, run rather more specialist medical courses of varying length, some leading to degrees.

Ideas for wives

In the hospital: teaching; cordon bleu for cooks; sewing lessons (and knitting); secretarial work; organising research projects. Helping in the various departments, especially pharmacy. Occupational and simple physiotherapy.

In the community: teaching; projects; weaving; beadwork; allotment; day old chicks. Nutritional education; organising a family planning programme. (Oxfam and other agencies will help with finance for a well thought out scheme.)

Agencies sending doctors/health workers to the third world

Name and address	Telephone
Action Health 2000, 33 Bird Farm Road, Fulbourn, Cambridge	0223 880194
AMREF (African Medical Research Foundation), 68 Upper Richmond Road, London SW15 2RP	01 874 4363
Britain-Nepal Medical Trust, Stafford House, 16 East Street, Tonbridge, Kent TN9 1HG	0732 365750
The British Red Cross Society, 9 Grosvenor Crescent, London SW1X 7ES	01 235 5454
Christians Abroad, 15 Tufton Street, London SW1P 3QQ	01 222 2165
Christian Medical Fellowship, 157 Waterloo Road, London SE1 8XN	01 928 4694
CIIR (Catholic Institute for International Relations), Overseas Volunteers, 22 Coleman Fields, London N1	01 354 0883
IVS (International Voluntary Service), Ceresole House, 53 Regent Road, Leicester LE1 6YL	0533 541862

100

Name and address	Telephone
ODA (Overseas Development Administration) Abercrombie House, Eaglesham Road, East Kilbride	03552 41199
OXFAM 274 Banbury Road, Oxford OX2 7DZ	0865 56777
Quaker Peace and Service Friends House, Euston Road, London NW1 2BJ	01 388 1977
Save The Children Fund Mary Datchelor House, 17 Grove Lane, Camberwell, London SE5 8RD	01 703 5400
Tear Fund 11 Station Road, Teddington, Middlesex TW11 9AA	01 977 9144
UNAIS (United Nations Association International Service) Recruitment, 3 Whitehall Court, London SW1A 2EL	930 0679/0
USPG (United Society for Propagation of Gospel) O/S Programmes, USPG House, 15 Tufton Street, Westminster, London SW1P 3QQ	01 222 4222
Volunteer Missionary Movement Shentey Lane, London Colney, Herts AL2 1AR	Bowmansgreen 24853
Voluntary Service Overseas 9 Belgrave Square, London SW1X 8PW	01 235 5191
World Vision of Europe 146 Queen Victoria Street, London EC4V 4BX	01 248 3056

List supplied by Bureau for Overseas Medical Service, London School of Hygiene and Tropical Medicine, Africa Centre, 38 King St, London WC2 8JT. Tel 01 836 5833.

Attend an inquest

R A B DRURY

"A true presentment make of all such matters and things. . . ."

The occasional attender at a coroner's court may feel that he has found in the inquest an unchanging aspect of our otherwise rapidly altering scene. But though the Victorian building may be the same as when you were a house surgeon—or even when your grandfather was—a light breeze of change has been blowing through the courtroom and its far older proceedings.

In 60 years the number of deaths reported to the coroner has more than doubled, but the number of inquests has fallen by a third. 1978 has seen the virtual disappearance of the coroner's jury following the implementation of one of the recommendations of the Brodrick Report.[1] The calling of a coroner's jury (part of whose oath is quoted above) is now an exceptional occasion for rare inquiries such as those into deaths in prison or fatal industrial accidents. With no jury, the occasional committal for manslaughter also becomes a thing of the past.

The absence of a jury has led to speedier completion of an inquest with less formality and no banging on doors, often in less august circumstances, since inquests may be held in many places such as offices or hospital committee rooms (but not on licensed premises). The cast and procedure remain largely unchanged, and those present will be the legally or medically (and sometimes both) qualified coroner, who will certainly have considerable knowledge and insight into the seamier side of medicine; his officer, usually a police officer with criminal investigation department experience, but sometimes a rural policeman at his first inquest; relatives of the deceased; one or more medical witnesses of the fact and cause of death; witnesses of the events leading to death; and others who will be called (occasionally subpoenaed) by the coroner's officer to attend.

Before the inquest

You will be told of the time, date, and place of the inquest. In

102

cases of unnatural or violent death necropsies are now universally carried out, and the clinician will know where, when, and by whom the necropsy will be performed. Attendance at this is desirable as both the clinician and the pathologist can learn much from each other, though their evidence will be independent and be based on their own observations at the bedside and in the postmortem room. With a knowledge of the circumstances leading to death and the findings at necropsy, the clinician should ask himself whether any complaint about lack of medical care could arise. In the event of this rare possibility a medical witness is a "proper interested party" who is entitled[2] to be legally represented at an inquest, and he should inform his medical defence organisation at once by telephone and be guided by them. If a doctor learns that relatives are to have legal representation, this does not automatically dictate that he should be legally represented unless he knows that criticisms are to be levelled at him. The vast majority of inquests have no such problems and the purpose is to inquire into the cause of death rather than matters of civil liability.

The clinician and pathologist should both be fully informed about the case before they attend the inquest because they will be asked questions of fact as well as of opinion. Retain the medical records of the patient and be familiar with the medical and nursing records as well as details of treatment. An incomplete grasp of the facts casts doubt on the validity of a witness's opinions.

At the inquest

It is not only courteous to the coroner and to the deceased's relatives to arrive in time and suitably dressed (not funereally attired), but also prudent, as many coroners take the medical evidence early and allow a doctor to leave if his evidence is not controversial. Make your arrival known to the coroner's officer and tell him if you wish to affirm rather than take the oath: the act of the renunciation of the Testament still causes a slight stir in the proceedings while a prearranged affirmation is accepted as a matter of course. In addition to the relatives, whom you will have met, and the pathologist, with whom you have already spoken, there may be solicitors acting for the deceased's family or other interested parties, and there will be one or more press reporters.

When your case starts you may be surprised at the informality of the proceedings. Coroner's courts are not bound by strict rules of evidence and the inquiry may include leading questions and hearsay evidence. Ensure that the court hears your evidence clearly and understands it, especially if names or diseases are unusual or difficult to spell. Speak in terms that can be understood by intelligent laymen, avoiding jargon. If details of rare clinical and pathological findings are necessary it is usually possible to lead up to these with a few explanatory words. There is always much consideration for the relatives, and in many inquests general medical findings are sufficient, with gruesome or harrowing medical evidence being avoided; likewise, coroners avoid publicising personal tragic details and suicide notes are seldom read out in full.

After your factual statements you will be questioned by the coroner, and possibly by solicitors or "properly interested parties." Usually it is possible to give straight answers, but medical witnesses are sometimes asked questions which they can answer only on hearsay evidence, if at all. If your reply is based on the observations of someone else, who is not in court, make this clear. Speak from memory with assurance, but refer to case records for details; avoid inaccuracies, however minor, as these may need correction later. An unexpected question impugning a lack of medical care is unlikely to be permitted by the coroner, or need not be answered. An allegation of negligence without warning can make a doctor a "properly interested person" and the coroner can allow him to put relevant questions to witnesses,[2] but doctors will normally prefer to seek an adjournment of the hearing to arrange legal representation.

In traumatic deaths a medical witness may be able to give a valuable opinion on the type and degree of violence that caused the fatal injuries. In addition, evidence of previous disease or disability that would have made the deceased more prone to an accident or susceptible to its consequences may be highly relevant to the coroner's inquiries and will be of interest to insurance companies. Pathologists will be asked to state the cause of death but may also be asked to comment on the circumstances leading to death and it is in these cases that a full understanding of the final illness is essential. Be prepared to sign a statement of the salient points of your evidence before you leave the court.

At the end of the inquest, have a word with the relatives, whose inarticulate gratitude for your unsuccessful efforts will be more rewarding than the coroner's officer's payment for your attendance. As you drive back to the land of the living you will appreciate that the roots of some of our recent social legislation, the recognition of hazards in industry and adverse reactions to drugs or the contraceptive pill spring from medical evidence given at coroner's inquests.

[1] *The Brodrick Report of the Committee on Death Certification and Coroners.* London: HMSO, 1971.
[2] *Coroner's Rules*, 1984; Rule 20 (I).

Give evidence

BERNARD KNIGHT

The witness box is commonly held to be the place which most doctors shun with distaste and even trepidation. Even so, an appearance in court as a medical witness need not be an ordeal if the doctor observes a few simple rules. This applies equally well to both criminal and civil cases in the crown courts and to a lesser extent in magistrate's courts and coroner's inquests, the latter having been dealt with in another chapter. Certain doctors, such as police surgeons and forensic pathologists, make such frequent visits to the witness box that it might be thought that they become immune to the tensions and pitfalls of the courts; nevertheless, they can just as easily come to grief if they ignore the basic precautions.

There has long been a facetious saying that the doctor in court should "dress up, stand up, speak up, and shut up," and there is considerable merit in this advice. The doctor in the witness box should dress like a professional person and not like a disc-jockey or lumberjack. Not only is a fairly sober suit more appropriate to the many cases in which there was a fatal outcome, but an opinion uttered by someone who at least looks like a medical expert will carry that much more conviction.

Similarly, as long as it falls well short of condescension or arrogance, a confident demeanour will add weight to the substance of the evidence. As to speaking up, if the doctor's evidence is worth hearing, it is pointless to have it mumbled and muttered. This tends to give the impression that the witness is so unsure of the substance of his testimony that he is reluctant to have it heard. Inaudibility will not only lengthen the proceeds but irritate judge and counsel.

As to "shutting up," there is a further well known saying that "if one open's one's mouth, one puts one's foot in it." Any amplification should be limited to the matter under discussion; the loquacious witness is a delight to opposing counsel, who will encourage the doctor to tie himself in knots with his own tongue.

Importance of original statement

These general matters apart, the most important part of giving evidence takes place not in the court itself but in the original circumstances which generate the evidence. More than any other single factor, it is the original statement given to the police or to a solicitor—sometimes months or even years earlier—that determines whether or not the doctor is to get a rough ride in the witness box. It is vital that this first statement—which is a formal declaration of the facts known to the witness and, where appropriate, his opinion on those facts—should be exactly what the doctor is prepared to say orally when he stands before the court.

Therefore, the doctor must decide at the outset what are the limits to which he is willing to testify. He must consider all aspects of the case and decide on the factual demarcation beyond which he is not prepared to step. He must be prepared to "put his mouth where his pen was" when the time of trial arrives. So often, in the security of his consulting room, a doctor will dash off a sweeping statement, drawing unwise and perhaps unwarranted conclusions and opinions. Then, when he is on his feet before a crowded court, the previous literary bravado tends to drain away and he fails to "come up to proof," as his legal colleagues would term it. In these circumstances not only will he do the court and justice a disservice, but he will almost certainly have a very uncomfortable time from opposing counsel and possibly the judge or magistrate. So often one has seen a barrister waving a sheaf of papers at the discomforted medical witness as he says, "But doctor, let me read what you said last February."

It cannot be overemphasised that the medical witness should never commit himself to opinions that he is not willing to maintain. This is not to say that he should never admit to being wrong in the face of new facts or interpretations from elsewhere, but he should not back off at the time of trial from his own earlier opinions.

Preparing the facts

The second necessity is the preparation of the facts. Whether he is attending as a witness to fact or as an expert witness with opinions, the medical witness should have done his homework sufficiently to be seen in the witness box to have at least an adequate grasp of the matters under discussion. Too often, the sorry sight is seen of a doctor standing sheepishly in the witness box, giving the impression that he has never heard of the person about whom he is being questioned and has no idea of any medical facts relating to the case. Under such circumstances, counsel becomes sarcastic and the judge himself incensed to the point of apoplexy. The doctor should bring all records relating to the patient; he should have read them beforehand; and he should refer to them when questioned, rather than mutter and stammer in a vain attempt to remember the relevant details. Such records must be originals, such as actual case notes or the contemporary reports made by the witness himself.

The use of such records in the witness box may have to be approved by the judge, who may wish to see them, to check that they are originals. He will always allow the doctor to refer to them for the purpose of "refreshing his memory," so that it is as well if the medical witness avoids shuffling them and searching as if this was the first time he had ever set eyes upon them.

Thirdly, the doctor should never trespass beyond the bounds of his own skill or competence. A junior house officer is not expected to give opinions which might tax the capabilities of a senior consultant—if he does so, he is likely to be destroyed by opposing counsel. Similarly, a senior specialist is equally vulnerable when he transgresses the boundaries of his own specialty. The classical example was the comment of Mr Alec Bourne, the well known gynaecologist, when Sir Bernard Spilsbury unwisely gave an opinion about clinical obstetrics. Mr Bourne said that, however eminent Sir Bernard was as a forensic pathologist, when he spoke of childbirth his evidence should be treated with contempt. The doctor who is pressed to answer questions which he considers to be beyond his sphere of skill should draw a firm line and indicate to the court—by appeal to the judge if necessary—that he feels unable to give a useful opinion.

Courtesy and consideration

The days of blood and thunder advocacy are thankfully past and counsel today are almost invariably courteous and considerate, especially to witnesses in a sister profession. Nevertheless, this does not detract from the penetrating intellect and piercing questions with which they can nail the medical witness to the courtroom wall. When the doctor has allowed himself to stray on to the thin ice of doubtful fact or the swampy ground of unwise opinion, the best course is to cut his losses and regain terra firma as gracefully as possible, by admitting that he does not know some fact or that he allows that a contrary opinion may be correct.

Whatever happens, embarrassment and loss of face should not tempt the doctor into anger, sarcasm, or even impertinence. Not only will this earn a rebuke from the judge, but it delights opposing counsel, who can run rings round an angry witness like a matador around a bewildered bull. Nevertheless, this state of affairs is rarely likely to happen if the doctor is well prepared, has kept within the perimeter of his original considered opinion, and gives his evidence and responses to questions calmly and responsibly.

There are two last points. Firstly, evidence needs to be given slowly and in short instalments, especially in the crown courts, as the judge will be writing it down longhand. Some doctors have suggested that the barrister who is on his feet suffers from intermittent catalepsy, but in reality he is watching the end of the judge's pen before putting the next question and the experienced medical witness will do the same. Secondly, the doctor should use comprehensible language in court, free from medical jargon. Even though the barristers and the judge may know almost as much about the medical aspects of the case as the doctor, the rest of the court—including the jury, if there is one—may not have the slightest idea of what the witness is talking about. From motives of sheer thoughtlessness, from professional pomposity, or even because a retreat into the familiar terminology is comforting during the uneasy vigil in the witness box, many doctors relapse into the jargon of our mysterious medical language. The good witness will translate his evidence into everyday English. Often the more junior doctors are the worst offenders; two of their classical gems are "periorbital haematomata" for "black eyes" and "biventricular myocardial hypertrophy" for "a big heart."

Raise funds

A K THOULD

"Can anyone remember when the times were not hard, and money not scarce?"—
RALPH WALDO EMERSON

Desperate times beget desperate remedies. When no money is available from conventional sources then there are only two courses open to you: either find funds by other means or give up in despair and take it out on your garden. However, if the project of your heart's desire still eats at your soul, then lesson one of fundraising is that if *you* are convinced that the enterprise is worthy and the plan is viable, don't let anyone put you off, and don't be disheartened because the country is bankrupt. It is never the right time to raise money, so go ahead and do it anyway.

Lesson two is that if you think fundraising is merely a matter of saying to yourself: "there are 300 000 people in this county, so if everyone gives 50p we will be home and dry"—forget it, go home, and tend your roses instead. Nobody is interested in handing over their hard earned cash unless you can convince them that the whole scheme is sound, necessary, and appealing to *them*. After all, why should they? Fundraising is grinding hard work. You must be prepared to kiss your wife and the baby goodbye for many evenings, because you will need to address any number of lay meetings. You will spend many hours at the kitchen table with your spouse signing letters and putting them in envelopes. You will go through agonies of self doubt and many crises of morale in your organisation. You will learn to endure the hunted look of your friends as they see you approach, hot with the news of your latest disaster or triumph. Fascinating for you; boring for them. If all this appears too much for you, with the seemingly endless hours of repetitive, slogging work, then don't go fundraising, not at any price—it is not for the faint-hearted.

Basic organisation

If you have lasted this far, and are still convinced of the rightness of your cause and the glamour of your appeal, then the next step is to set up your basic organisation. First of all, you will need a small but select band of trusted (voluntary) and dedicated hard-working helpers. You *must* have a very good secretary/typist, because you are going to need to send out a great many letters: thousands will be needed for a major appeal. Next, you need to gather together a small committee you can trust. The members will need to be long-suffering, industrious but enthusiastic, and, if possible, experienced in this sort of thing. They should, if possible, be well known and respected in the community, with many contacts in the business and professional worlds. Do not have a big committee. I suggest about ten as the maximum. You will need a good solicitor, because he will set up your trust and do the legal work—for nothing, if you're lucky. You must have a good, painstaking treasurer, used to handling large amounts of money without getting nightmares, and able to keep proper accounts. Above all, you must have a good, decent chairman, well known in the area at large, and carrying with him or her the aura of trust.

You ought to be the secretary yourself, and be prepared to do the dog work of arranging the committee business. You will need a bank account, and all cheques must be signed by the treasurer and yourself. Next you must get your solicitor to set your organisation up as a charitable trust. The procedure is tedious, but not particularly difficult, and be prepared for the Charity Commissioners to ask some searching and highly pertinent questions. When drawing up the articles of the trust, be sure you look ahead, so that you can continue to raise funds by way of the organisation in the future and can, within the articles, pursue whatever long-term projects you wish. Your solicitor will advise you. If you are successful, you will be given a number, and you must quote this in all your correspondence. If you don't, some charitable trusts may not be prepared to give you money.

Where to start

It is a good idea to start with a meeting to which you invite all the heads of the known fundraising organisations in your area, that is, the Women's Institute, Rotary Clubs, Lions, and so on. You will be surprised how many there are; you must find out who they are from your committee and local contacts, then draw up a list. Have your meeting in the early evening and provide sherry and whatnots to eat, but don't be too lavish. They will be looking for evidence that the money you raise goes to the appeal, not towards wasteful window dressing. Try not to be mean, however—the balance is important. Make up a brochure setting out your aims and objectives. Not glossy and expensively produced, but workmanlike and readable. A small book on the subject is unnecessary and will not be read. It needs to be short, informative, and to the point. Most of all, when someone asks you to go and give a talk on your project, then go, however inconvenient, and go at their time and convenience. Be prepared to answer questions and, above all, be honest and frank. If you feel your project needs a million pounds, then say so. The dissembler is soon mercilessly exposed and rightly so. Never underestimate your audience or talk down to them. They are probably more experienced at the game than you are. They are usually hard-headed but great-hearted people, and they need to be convinced of the essential worthiness and practicality of what you are doing.

Some fundraisers prefer to set up a local organisation of ardent supporters of the cause. If your project is a large one then this may be a sensible course. An effective way is to divide up your parish into districts and appoint a local committee for each district under a suitable leader. However, these district leaders need to be chosen with care. Enthusiasm is a necessary attribute, but good organisational ability, staying power, and the ability to lead and encourage but not bludgeon people are equally vital properties. A good district committee can safely be left to get on with local fundraising efforts. You will need to show regular and highly visible interest in their efforts, however, and regular coordination meetings are essential.

A further step is to get from the public library the published list of registered charities (there may be a waiting list to get it), then go through the three or four thousand listed there and see which ones may be interested in your cause. Write them a short letter setting out the facts and enclosing your brochure. About 95% of them will throw your application in the wastepaper basket. The other 5% may give you some money. If you can, and they will let you, offer to go and see their trustees in person.

Some recommend trying to raise money from the top thousand companies, but I have found this a waste of time. Only local industry seems to be interested in contributing to local causes, and this is all that one can expect. If there is a large industrial combine or combines near you, write to the managing director and go and see him. He will usually be courteous and give you a fair hearing. Just possibly, he may even advise his company to give you some money. Local businesses may be reached by looking them up in the yellow pages of the telephone directory; then write them a letter.

The letters themselves are important. They can be printed, using your appeal's logo at the head, but you must personally enter the name of the person you are writing to, and sign it personally.

This will mean signing many hundreds of letters, possibly thousands. If you are not prepared to give the personal touch, then don't expect to get much money. Nothing is worse than the cold, printed impersonal letter. It looks as if you are not prepared to take trouble, and, if you don't sign it yourself, this is probably true.

You must be prepared to go to endless donkey derbys, band festivals, sponsored walks, fêtes, and whatever. After all, if they are prepared to go to that much trouble to raise money for you, the least you can do is turn up, and make a short speech of thanks. Anyway, it is all enormous fun for most of the time.

Publicity and costs

The local press will probably be interested and, in my experience, helpful, but they like to be kept informed of how things are going. In return, they will give you a few column inches of publicity at intervals. Be careful, however, about self advertisement. It is a good idea to check with the Medical Defence Union about how far you can go. Almost any publicity is valuable, unless your treasurer makes off with the funds. It is worth asking to have a stand at the local county show—they will probably give you a site at cheap rates.

Costs should be kept to less than 1% of the money you raise, so spend as little as you can on your organisation. Your worst expense will be on postage—the costs of printing should be relatively trivial (use the office roneo). Car stickers are worthwhile and cheap—if you can persuade people to display them. The Charity Commissioners will expect you to have your accounts properly audited and these must be readily available. So keep good records; don't be like Samuel Johnson, who observed that he had two very cogent reasons for not printing any list of subscribers—one that he had lost all the names; the other that he had spent all the money.

When it is all over, invite your subscribers to see what their money has bought, and be generous in your thanks. Do not forget to announce that your fundraising appeal is now over, at least for the time being; otherwise people may go on raising unnecessary funds for you to the detriment of other equally worthy appeals whose turn it now is. The reward for you will be the immense satisfaction of seeing your project completed. It will have been very hard going and at times discouraging, but the glow of satisfaction is very warm. Good luck.

Apply for a research grant

JAMES HOWIE

Success in applying for a research grant depends on producing clear evidence of a good question that needs to be answered; of a capacity to make a promising attempt at finding the answer; of reasonable opportunity to do the work in good conditions and within a defined period; and of the need for specified finance for stated purposes. The application will be read and assessed by experienced, sceptical officials—lay and scientific—and by chosen assessors—usually senior academics who have a good knowledge of the subject and a capacity for fair and reliable judgment of people and proposals. Answers to applications are seldom available in under three months; and it may take much longer, depending on dates of meetings, and whether the application is clear or vague (in which case the applicant may be asked to provide supplementary information). In some circumstances delays of six months are quite reasonable; applicants should allow plenty of time, and find out from the grant-giving body the best date for submitting an application. Usually a standard application form has to be completed, and this should always be clearly typed, and suitable for copying. If the form does not allow enough space for a full answer under any of its headings, submit an appendix and indicate that you have done this by a note at the corresponding place on the form.

A good question to be answered

One of the distinguishing attributes of a good research worker is his ability to find good questions to be answered. A good question is one whose answer will matter. It may matter because it clarifies a fundamental issue of medical or pure science, or affects medical practice in some appreciable way. The answer must advance knowledge or understanding, which means that it must be more than a mere footnote. It must convey positive information.

113

Negative findings, however useful to others working on the same subject, are not of themselves a good complete answer. Nor is it enough simply to provide an account of new methods for doing things without showing that the results mean something. "I'm not interested in recipes—only in puddings," said one leading assesor. So the applicant must identify the question to be answered and specify it in a clear and understandable way, quoting briefly the immediately relevant work on the same subject.

Capacity to answer the question

Inspirations drawn out of the air, even by the most ingenious minds, seldom appeal to sceptical assessors. But if the applicant has a new thought about a long unanswered question he has made a good start. Some people have found useful problems by reading three or four standard textbooks to discover statements that have obviously been copied from one book to another, and that are generally accepted as truth without having been properly tested in modern times. A good piece of observation of some unexpected finding during routine work is an excellent starting point, even if it is not by itself enough to make the basis of an application for a grant. It is almost essential to do, and preferably to publish, some unaided work on the chosen topic. If it can be given to and criticised by a scientific meeting, so much the better. This unaided work establishes that you have a valid starting point, that you stand on some foundation, and that you have some initiative and motivation. Grant-giving bodies, like wise generals, prefer to reinforce success, however modest, rather than to give money hoping that some purely armchair strategy may lead to a real advance.

There are no good questions on which an able research worker cannot make some progress without outside help. Evidence of motivation, initiative, and capacity are what assessors look for; and nothing is better evidence that they are backing a likely winner than proof that the horse has already jumped a few fences and knows what lies ahead. Those who are beginners at research, in the sense that their work is not yet well known, must always supply a curriculum vitae as well as saying what their problem is and how they hope to tackle it. The same information is required about any named collaborators still unknown to the grant-giving body. This kind of information is normally given in appendices.

Opportunity for work and evidence of need

Unknown applicants need to prove that they have the necessary accommodation and basic facilities for the work proposed. Usually these will be found in an established university department, good hospital, or practice whose head is known as a supervisor of research, and who supports the application in writing. Unknown applicants should not expect the grant-giving body to build or find accommodation for them, or to buy basic equipment such as microscopes, centrifuges, and laboratory furniture. Yet these are often asked for, and such requests cool the welcome given to the application.

Specialised apparatus and highly qualified technical help may be given as part of a grant, but only to workers of proved capacity and then only if they can show that the apparatus is essential, not reasonably to be provided for the applicant's ordinary work, and fully and accurately costed, preferably with manufacturer's specifications and quotations in support. Such information should go in appendices.

Duration of the research

How much time will the work require? And what will happen to the applicant and any collaborators when it is finished? With money hard to find for research, or for any advanced work, grant-giving bodies must ask these questions before deciding on which grants to support. Those who can live indefinitely and happily as full-time research workers are not all that numerous; so it is an advantage to see as clearly as possible what the applicant and his collaborators expect to live on when the grant runs out. Some, indeed, will adopt careers as full-time research workers; but these are in a minority. So it helps to have at least the prospect of an established post when the grant ends.

It is also necessary to show a plan of work that may be expected to supply some sort of answer in three years at the most. This, in turn, may lead to an extension; but the grant-giving body must be shown that there is a sensible plan—statistically assessed from the beginning, if possible—to guarantee that the necessary observations can be made within the time from the material available, and that they will be competently documented in such a way that they may be analysed. Even if the answer is a lemon, the work should be so planned that even this harsh truth will be clear within reasonable time. Nothing is more chilling to grant-giving bodies than the fear that they are about to support an expedition into never-never land to discover goodness knows what.

A last word

How do you know that your idea is a good one? Well, you don't know; and neither does the grant-giving body. If you did know the answer in advance, the work would be too dull to be worth doing. But there are some obvious bits of applied work crying out for a yes or no answer, and it's not a bad idea to join a team on one of these projects just to see if you feel the genuine thrill of doing research—any research. Also, if you suddenly have a feeling that you're on to something so urgent and so obviously right that you're bound to have the answer in six weeks at the most, while it lasts you will have a single-minded obsession and happiness that cannot be surpassed; and you are probably at the start of something that will really matter. It may well destroy your original hypothesis; but it will probably keep you busy for years to come.

Plan a research project

M D WARREN

Disciplined inquiry, review of current practice, and research are components of the practice of medicine. Each of these activities requires detailed planning and the writing of a protocol, which may form the basis of an application for a research grant, and will be the yardstick for the measurement of progress and achievement in the project. The protocol should set out the aims of the project, how these are to be achieved, how bias will be eliminated, the subjects or types of patients to be studied, the ethical aspects, and the proposed statistical analysis. It should establish that the expenditure of effort, time, and money is likely to be worth while. Planning and statistical advice should be sought at the preliminary stages of the study.

The questions and suggestions listed below are intended as an aide-mémoire for those planning a research project, whether this is to be a descriptive study, a clinical trial, or a survey.

Aide-mémoire for preparing a protocol

(1) *What is the purpose of the study?*

What are the aims and precise objectives? What questions are to be answered? Is the purpose to test, examine, or evaluate current practice or a new treatment, procedure, or service or to obtain new facts about the causation or natural history of a disease?

(2) *What is already known about the problem?*

What are the gaps in present knowledge? How will the proposed study contribute to our knowledge and understanding of the problem?

(3) *Is the proposal a pilot or main study?*

(4) *What design will be used in the project?*

Will the study be basically a laboratory project, a clinical trial or a survey? Will it be a trial of an "intervention"—for example, a treatment, procedure, or service (therapeutic, preventative, caring, or educational)? Will it be a case-control study with randomised or matched controls or a quasi-experimental study? If a survey, will it be conducted by questionnaire, interview, or clinical examination? Will it be retrospective, cross-sectional, or prospective (cohort)? Is a "blind" or "double-blind" design proposed?

(5) *How are the subjects of the study to be chosen?*

What is the population from which the subjects will be drawn (the denominator in incidence and prevalence studies)? Are the subjects of the study the total population of a community or all patients with a certain diagnosis? What are the entry and exclusion criteria for choosing subjects? How are the controls to be chosen? Will a sample of the total population or of all potential subjects be examined? If so, how is a sample to be obtained to ensure that it is representative of the total population? Attention must be paid to the definition of the criteria for selection, to the sampling methods, and to the number of subjects needed to obtain a significant result.

(6) *What data are to be collected, and why?*

What factors (variables) are already thought to affect the outcome? What factors contained in the new hypothesis are being tested? What factors (if present) might distort the representativeness of the results? What are the indicators or measures of the outcomes of the trial or experiment? The amount of data collected should be limited, though measures of different dimensions of outcome should be used when possible.

(7) *What are the treatment schedules or other activities forming the "intervention" in the study, and how are the variables to be defined and measured?*

The techniques, dosage, programmes of treatment, prophylaxis, other activities, etc, must be standardised; this is especially important in multicentre studies. Explicit decisions must be taken about how the presence or absence of disease is to be determined (for example, hypertension and diabetes), how severity and duration are to be measured, and how social and demographic variables are to be defined and measured (for example, marital state, occupation, and social class). If possible, the proposed definitions and measurements should be consistent with those used in comparable studies; if they are not, the reasons for the differences should be stated.

(8) *How are the data to be collected and the measurements to be made?*

Have the methods been tested? Are they valid (that is, do they actually measure what they are intended to)? Are they reliable (that is, can they be repeated to yield the same results)? Are they sensitive (that is, can they identify all positive cases)? Are they specific (that is, can they identify only positive cases)? Will data be collected by observation, examination, interview, or from record forms? Will special recording forms be needed? Who will collect the data? What training will they need? Should an independent observer make the baseline or outcome measurements (or both)? What checks and controls will be used to maintain accuracy and objectivity?

(9) *How will the data be processed and analysed?*

Will this be done by computer or some other method? Must the data be coded and punched on to cards? If so, who will do this? How will the analysis proceed? How will the data be presented? What form of report is likely to result?

(10) *What problems of ethics and etiquette does the project raise?*

Are patients' rights properly observed? How are the consent and collaboration of patients, interviewees, doctors, nurses, social workers, and others to be obtained? How is the confidentiality of the data to be ensured? What agreements are to be made about publication? Has the project been approved by the ethics committee?

(11) *What arrangements are to be made for creating or referring patients for whom new needs come to light as a result of the project?*

Can the local services cope? Or will special arrangements be needed?

(12) *What is the expected timetable for the study?*

In what order will the different stages of the investigation be carried out? It is helpful to set out what is to be done and by whom in chronological order with estimates of the duration of each activity. Enough time should be allowed for analysing the data and preparing the report (that is, the presentation, synthesis, and interpretation of the raw data).

(13) *What will the project cost?*

What will be the cost in manpower, including the time of the main investigator? What will be the cost of capital equipment? What will be the cost of additional salaries (plus pension and National Insurance contributions), rent for accommodation, travelling and subsistence, stationery, printing, postage, telephone, photocopying, administrative costs, and overheads? What outside help and advice will be needed, and how much will it cost? What is already available? What additional resources are required?

Sources of funds

There are a number of sources of funds available for the support of research. Within the National Health Service district health authorities and some postgraduate medical centres may be able to give grants to cover expenses for materials, postage, and clerical assistance, but not usually for salaries of research staff. Since 1958 there has been a scheme for research funding operated by the regional health authorities. This scheme, known as the locally organised research scheme is intended to support research by medical, nursing, and paramedical staff and others working in the scientific and technical services of the NHS. General practitioners and professional staff working in community health services are eligible for grants. Grants can be given for studies on the prevention, cause or treatment of disease, on methods of caring for patients in the community as well as in the hospitals, and on epidemiological investigations and studies of health services when these can be undertaken with relatively modest support. DHSS health circulars HSC (75) 148, 1975 and HC (78) 10, 1978 set out the details. The DHSS, through the office of the chief scientist makes substantial grants for research not only through its support for research units and programmes, but also for one off projects. The office of the chief scientist has set up a small grants committee, which considers spontaneous research proposals in the areas of health and personal social services research which cost up to £44 000 (in 1983) and are of no more than three years' duration. The DHSS publishes each year a *Handbook of Research and Development* in which all research funded by the office of the chief scientist is listed and indications are given in the publication of priority areas for funding. Whilst the DHSS is principally concerned with applied research and the many facets of health

120

services research, the Medical Research Council and the Economic and Social Research Council fund more basic research. Although the emphasis of the MRC is on clinical and biological research, it does now fund health services research. Outside the DHSS and the NHS there are many grant-giving bodies ranging from the large national institutions such as the Nuffield Provincial Hospitals Trust and the King's Fund to organisations concerned with research into particular diseases and patient groups (for guidance, see *Handbook of the Association of Medical Research Charities*, 1983, and *Research Funds Guide*, 3rd edition, British Medical Association, 1976).

Applicants for research funds may be required to complete a detailed application form. Such a form must be completed fully and in the manner prescribed. Research committees are not impressed by applicants who do not take meticulous trouble over their submissions. If an applicant wishes to provide additional information, this should be done on separate sheets and referred to in the appropriate place on the form. The applicant should enquire from the funding body whether there is a particular date by which applications must be received. Some research advisory committees meet annually, some twice a year and some quarterly, so that to miss a meeting can postpone the start of a project by many months. Most committees seek the views of specialist referees about the design and worthwhileness of a proposed study, so a protocol should be written with this in mind.

Further reading

Abramson, J H. *Survey methods in community medicine*, 3rd Ed. London: Churchilll Livingstone, 1984.

Alderson, M, and Dowie, R. *Health surveys and related studies. Reviews of United Kingdom statistical sources vol IX*. Oxford: Pergamon Press, 1979.

Barker, D J P, and Rose, G. *Epidemiology in medical practice*, 2nd Ed. London: Churchill Livingstone, 1979.

Calnan, J. *One way to do research. The A-Z for those who must*. London: Heinemann, 1976.

Cancer Research Campaign Working Party, *Trials and tribulations: thoughts on the organisation of multicentre clinical studies. Br Med J* 1980; **281**: 918–20.

Cartwright, A. *Health surveys in practice and potential. A critical review of their scope and methods*. London: King's Fund Publishing Office, 1983.

Clinical Trials Unit, Department of Pharmacology and Therapeutics, London Hospital Medical College, *Aide-mémoire for preparing clinical trial protocols. Br Med J* 1977; i: 1323–4.

Goldstone, L A. *Understanding medical statistics*. London: Heinemann Medical Books, 1983.

Gore, S M. *Assessing clinical trials: trial size. Br Med J* 1981; **282**: 1687–9.

Hoinville, G, and Jowell, R. *Survey research practice*. London: Heinemann Educational Books, 1978.

Lock, S. *Thorne's better medical writing*. London: Pitman Medical, 1977.

Medical Research Council, *Responsibility in the use of medical information for research*. London: Medical Research Council, 1973.

Pocock, S J. *Clinical trials: a practical approach*. Chichester and New York: John Wiley, 1983.

Swinscow, T D V. *Statistics at square one*, 4th ed. London: British Medical Association, 1978.

Talk to a reporter

TONY SMITH

Doctors are mostly ambivalent about the press, radio, and television. Sometimes a series of articles or TV programmes appears which explains a new technical advance clearly, accurately, and with sensible, informed speculation about its future implications. On these occasions doctors join the mass audience in admiring the skill and imagination of the team responsible. But doctors also remember programmes and articles which distorted the truth in the pursuit of sensationalism—BBC's *Panorama* on brain death remaining the outstanding example. Sometimes, too, when a new technique has caught the public imagination there may be a siege of a hospital with reporters competing for exclusive rights to interview patients or their relatives—and some using lies and confidence trickery in an attempt to extract confidential information from hospital staff.

Of course the public has a legitimate interest in hearing about medical advances, and often the best way for the story to be presented is with a "human interest" angle; but most doctors have heard horror stories about smooth-talking reporters who try to discover the identity of a patient who has a right to privacy, and many fear that if they talk to the press they may find an incautious comment given headline treatment.

Ask for time

How, then, should a doctor respond when his telephone rings and he finds a reporter (from the press, radio, or TV) wanting to talk about a news story—either an incident concerning a particular patient or a technical advance of some kind? My first piece of advice is to ask for time. Few of us are practised enough at public speaking to think on our feet, and I find it invaluable to ask for a few minutes to put my thoughts together. In fact, I usually make a few notes of what I want to say. A 10–20 minute pause will give

122

you time to check a few facts (what exactly is the incubation period of mumps?), possibly have a quick chat with a colleague, and, if you are in any doubt, to take advice. (What sort of advice? You may want to ask your hospital secretary whether he is issuing a press statement, and if so would he prefer doctors to refer all callers to him; or you may wish to discuss confidentiality with your defence society. If there is any possibility of litigation you should almost certainly say nothing without having first checked with the legal experts.)

So after 10 minutes the reporter rings back. At this point you may have decided to make no comment either on legal advice or because the subject (such as, say, artificial insemination by donor in lesbians) is one which you'd prefer to avoid for fear of getting egg on your face. Don't explain why; simply apologise for wasting his time and say that having had time to think you have decided not to comment. Mostly, however, you'll want to do what you can to answer the questions. But next find out on what basis you are talking. Is the reporter simply seeking background information, talking off the record? Is he wanting attributable statements that will appear (or be heard) with your name attached? Or is he sounding you out for a possible interview on TV or radio? The distinction is important, and it is up to you to ask, not the reporter to explain. If he is asking you for attributable comments on a news story then you should ask him to read out exactly what is going to be printed. If he tells you that he is still putting the story together, then ask him to phone you later with the final version, including your comment, to make sure that it still sounds right in context.

Studio punch-ups

He may be wanting you to come and talk in a sound or TV studio. Karl Sabbagh explains how TV features are made. In general, my advice on the studio punch-ups with a doctor, a lawyer, a sociologist, a trade union official, two coalminers, and a dog is—leave them to the experts. Talking one-to-one with a reporter is fair enough; multipanel discussions usually leave the participants angry and frustrated.

On the whole, however, talking to reporters can be fun—intellectually stimulating and worth while. But please don't talk about something outside your range of current knowledge—what you learnt about virology in medical school is not good enough 12 years later. Don't criticise another doctor's treatment—he's seen the patient and you haven't. Don't say that anyone concerned is a fool unless you've met him or her and you're certain. Don't seem to assume that patients are invariably ignorant, lazy, and wrong and that doctors are always conscientious, polite, considerate, and right. And don't answer any questions you don't want to answer.

Then, with any luck, you'll get to know your reporter and he'll come to you again and learn to rely on you—and you on him. Once that occurs you'll be able to forget all the horror stories.

Give a press conference

PAMELA TAYLOR

Never call a press conference if you can cover all the information in a written press statement or by telephoning the newspapers. Journalists will not thank you for calling them away from their desks unnecessarily.

A press conference must be planned, whether you have weeks of time or the journalists are milling around outside the door. Your check list should be:

The invitation	Personnel
Timing	The conference
Invitation list	Photographers
Venue	TV and radio
Badges and signing in	Picking up the pieces

The invitation

Depending on the event, you may send embossed cards for a formal conference, issue a written invitation, ring round frantically giving an hour or so's notice, or call out, as the press jostle you, that you will be commenting in the Hospital Board Room in twenty minutes.

For the embossed card, formal event give the journalists plenty of warning. Send the press a covering letter giving fuller details and remember to inform them about dress.

A written press invitation should contain enough information to encourage the journalists to attend. Once written, your invitation may be hot news, so put an embargo (figure) on it for the time of the conference.

Time may be too short for written invitations. Jot down the essential details, grab some volunteers, and ring round the journalists or their newsdesks.

125

> PLEASE DO NOT BROADCAST OR PUBLISH IN ANY FORM
> BEFORE 11.30 AM THURSDAY 13TH OCTOBER 1984

Embargo notice for the invitation.

Timing

A good time for a press conference is 11.30 am, giving the journalists time to write up their stories afterwards, before their late afternoon deadlines. Make special arrangements to meet deadlines for evening and local newspapers and magazines; you can brief them in advance under embargo, so they can write the bulk of their stories and attend the conference for quotes and the finishing touches.

Any day of the week will do, but a Friday conference will make Saturday's papers, which have lower circulations. Weekend conferences are not unknown, but the daily press work on Sundays, not Saturdays, and the Sunday newspapers will want some convincing to give you space at short notice.

Invitation list

Draw up a list of those journalists you and your colleagues know and invite them by name. Then compile a list of the remaining publications and send invitations to their newsdesks.

Invite press representatives from as many relevant publications as you can. There are paramedical and scientific journals, local newspapers, national press, independent and BBC radio and television. Resist considering a publication or a programme from one of these categories as unsuitable to invite. The journalist is the best judge of what the public wants.

Invitation lists for press conferences called on the spot are out of the question. Round up the press who are milling around and ask someone to telephone quickly any special press contacts you have.

Venue

The success of a major public relations event will depend heavily on the venue. Many conference centres and hotels provide good facilities and staff trained to try to cope with your every need. Bear in mind transport facilities, car parking, and hotel accommodation for out of town sites, and catering and visual aids.

The best place to hold a news press conference is on your own premises. You need a room, a table and chairs for the speakers, and enough chairs facing them for the journalists. Make sure you know where the nearest telephone is, and the nearest typewriter. Prop up some name plates in front of the speakers, even if they are written in felt tip on plain cardboard. Tea or coffee is appreciated on arrival and you may run to refreshments afterwards.

Badges and signing in

It is useful to give journalists badges so everyone knows who they are talking to. Journalists can be checked off against a list of acceptances and given badges with their names and publications. On less formal occasions journalists can write their own names on stick-on badges. Don't waste time on badges for a hurried press conference. Just ask them all to sign in; a sheet of paper with two columns headed "name" and "representing" will do. A record of attendance is useful if a resulting story needs following up; it also helps you build up a press list, and check numbers for the catering bill.

Personnel

The setpiece conference needs a programme for the chairman's welcome, Minister's or other guest's contribution, any film, and questions. Often, a press conference is a time when the person at the top puts in a rare appearance, giving an over-long speech. When you know you are dealing with such an event, give timings in your invitation so the journalists know what they are in for. Invite enough staff to keep the show running smoothly and brief them on the special responsibilities of talking to the press.

The final choice of speakers is often dictated by internal politics, rows behind the scenes and, occasionally, common sense. Ideally, the most senior person with a detailed knowledge of the subject should be present. Add a chairman, essential for keeping control, and perhaps one other person with specialist knowledge.

However short of time you are, a rehearsal is essential. You must know who is to cover which aspects of the information to be given and how questions are to be dealt with.

The conference

Introductions from the chairman should be followed by short speeches from the participants. Speeches and any audiovisual material should be kept to the minimum necessary to explain the position. Avoid inphrases, abbreviations, and jargon. If you are reading from a prepared statement let the press have copies; this helps them report you accurately.

The style of press conference will dictate the type of written material given out. Speeches typed up or photocopied from handwritten notes, will be enough for a news conference, but photographs, biographical details of the speakers, diagrams, and background material may also be made available at the time, or in advance under embargo. If you are launching a publication, detailed report, or the results of research work an easily understood synopsis should be made available.

Take all questions at the end. During questions never openly disagree with your fellow participants; correct something said tactfully. Tell the truth and don't try to dodge any questions. If you don't know an answer, say so.

Photographers

Photographers invite themselves without warning. They stand in the front and pop electronic flash guns in your face. You may wish to limit numbers by providing a photographer of your own who will make arrangements to supply all the interested publications, meeting their various deadlines.

Photographers door stepping are a fact of press relations life. If you take part in delegations of national interest or announce major medical advances, you must expect to be photographed.

TV and radio

Television interviews and their crews need advance warning.

Special consideration must be given to the requirements of both television and radio journalists who will have to sit anxiously through the press conference watching their looming deadlines. There may be time to record a quick interview before the press conference, but the journalists will not want to be kept waiting while you give the BBC special treatment.

After the press conference, make sure there is a quiet place you can escape to for interviews. This is particularly important for radio, which, unlike television, cannot record a quick sentence or two out on the pavement.

Record the interviews according to deadlines. The work can be shared if more than one person took part in the press conference.

You may be asked to go to the studios to record an interview, or appear live. Tell them to send a car to pick you up, and to take you on afterwards.

Picking up the pieces

Planned follow up to a press conference is essential.

Immediately following the conference, during any refreshments, in the corridor, or over the telephone go over points with individual journalists, particularly if you did not handle a question well during the conference.

Check the press coverage and clear up any errors or differences of opinion, either by submitting a letter for publication, or having a word with the journalist, asking for your particular point to be included next time the subject is written on.

Remember, you will be competing for column inches and air time with many others, and, despite all the advice, there is no guarantee of success.

Become a medical journalist or editor

STELLA LOWRY, RICHARD SMITH

We have been prompted to write this article by the increasing numbers of medical students and doctors contacting the *BMJ* (and presumably other medical publications) asking about a career in medical journalism or editing. Yet we doubt if even one of the seven million people who have been to medical schools since the dawn of time has gone with the idea of becoming a medical journalist or editor.

Those handful of doctors who do become medical journalists or editors usually decide to follow this strange path after they have graduated and for some very practical reason—such as that they are broke, can't get any other sort of a job, or are fed up of being a round peg in a square hole. They usually have literary leanings or pretensions, are divergent thinkers, and, as Dr Tony Smith, deputy editor of the *BMJ*, puts it, "have some sort of wooden leg." But medical journalism is not just a refuge for broken down doctors, and Sarah Jenkins, editor of *Medical News*, said to us: "All too often those doctors seeking jobs in medical journalism are dissatisfied with medical practice and are seeking alternative ways of making a living but have no real commitment to journalism." This is an important piece of advice: If you're simply looking for a way out of clinical medicine and have no real interest in editing or journalism then try something else.

We have been conscious that much of the advice we give to people who come to see us has been ragged and disorganised (and to some extent this is inevitable because medical journalism is a ragged and disorganised business, and therein lies much of its pleasure and heartache), and we thought we would try to bring together our suggestions. In preparing the article we wrote to several editors of medical publications and asked them how many doctors they employ, what the doctors do, and how many vacancies they will have in the next five years. Their answers are summarised in the table.

130

What do medical journalists do?

Plenty of schoolchildren climb on the conveyor belt that turns them into doctors with only a hazy idea of what being a doctor entails, and it is when the belt delivers them into disagreeable and unforseen circumstances that their minds turns to journalism. So we hope that they will not repeat their mistakes and will try to find out more about what it is like to be a medical journalist or editor. They will find this difficult because medical journalists are a small and heterogeneous group. One or two make much of their money writing colourful articles for colourful lay publications; the odd one here and there is a medical correspondent for a national newspaper; some write potboilers; and some write literature; but most plug away editing and writing for medical publications that are read mostly by other (and proper) doctors.

A distinction must be drawn between being a journalist and being an editor. The doctors who work for the *BMJ*, the *Lancet*, and other scholarly publications spend most of their time editing—that is, selecting papers for publication and preparing those that are selected. People who want to be creative and who "really want to write novels" will not be happy sifting through piles of complicated papers, arguing with dissatisfied authors, and fretting over whether a colon should really be a semi-colon. As Dr Stephen Lock, editor of the *BMJ*, says: "We at the *BMJ* are mostly just taking in other people's washing."

Those who want to express themselves will probably be better employed seeking their fortune as journalists—people who write what they want, concern themselves little or not at all with the writings of others, and have subeditors to turn the ungrammatical but inspiring into the grammatical and slightly less inspiring. Medical newspapers, such as *Medical News*, *Pulse*, and *General Practitioner*, employ doctors as journalists, and some offer a training. And once your foot is in the door, you have dashed off a few pieces, and your word processor bristles with contacts then you can launch into a profitable freelance career.

Something that all those who contemplate metamorphosing from doctor to journalist should remember is that doctors (believe it or not) are highly regarded by most people in Britain, whereas journalists (and editors are rightly tarred with the same brush) rank no better than politicians and union leaders and are thought of as mendacious, unfeeling, greedy, and drunken. In reality, of course, there are just as many wicked doctors as journalists, but this sudden drop in status may put some aspiring journalists off while it may positively attract others.

Getting your foot in the door

Many of those who come to see us at the *BMJ* don't want to hear our ideas on what medical journalists and editors do; they simply want to know how they can become one. This is obviously a problem when there are only a few jobs: they don't become available often and when they do you may miss the advertisement. (All of the publications we spoke to, except *World Medicine*, advertise in the medical press.) One way round the problem of not being in the right place at the right time is to make yourself known to medical editors. Hustling is part of the stock in trade of journalists, and you may get a free lunch if not a career. Obviously, however, if more and more doctors contemplate turning journalist then editors will grow tired of being approached, and the very fact that we are writing this article suggests that we are some way down that path.

The table gives some idea of what editors say they are looking for in applicants for jobs. But we suspect that what counts most is some indefinable pazazz and a feeling on the editor's part that he could bare being locked up with you in a small office for several years. Wide medical experience is said by almost all the editors to be important, and so it is, but many successful medical editors and journalists are thin on both postgraduate qualifications and medical experience. It is impossible to say what use a training in journalism would be because we know of no medical journalists who have had a training before applying for a job. Such a training shouldn't count against you (although in such a fickle world it might), but most editors say they would prefer more medical experience.

Something that will undoubtedly impress editors is having had something (and preferably lots) published. Even an article (but not a portrait) in the *Sun* will count a little, but two articles in *Nature*, a five page essay in the *New England Journal of Medicine*, and a first review in the *Times Literary Supplement* will impress much more. (A book of poetry we suggest you keep to yourself.) Getting into print is not difficult, and even swallowing rejections will do you nothing but good. So if you do fancy a career in medical journalism reading and writing a lot and sending articles off to publications will be useful. Editing the medical school magazine may also help, although most editors don't seem to be much impressed by this achievement.

Looking abroad

Another way round the problem of there being only a few openings might be to look abroad. In France, for instance, most of the medical correspondents for national newspapers are qualified doctors, but we doubt if many British graduates will have a good enough grasp of French to earn their living in that language. More sensibly and traditionally, they will look to other English speaking countries, which means in this context the United States, Canada, and Australia (all the other countries are too small to employ doctors full time as editors or journalists).

Both the *Journal of the American Medical Association* and the *Canadian Medical Association Journal* have fellowship programmes for doctors who want to train as editors. The American one is called the Fishbein fellowship and it started in 1978. We wrote to Dr Alan Blum for more information about openings in North America and Australasia. He was a Fishbein fellow and was editor of the *Medical Journal of Australia* before becoming editor of the *New York State Journal of Medicine*. He tells us that a Fishbein fellow works as an editor on *JAMA*, reviewing papers, attending editorial meetings, and writing short pieces and reports on conferences. Dr Blum thinks that the fellowship provides an outstanding opportunity.

One problem for a British graduate is that these fellowships naturally tend to go to Americans and Canadians, but Dr Blum holds out an olive branch for British students: he has started a 10 week summer research assistantship at the *New York State Journal of Medicine* and says he will be delighted to consider British applicants. (We are also considering such an assistantship for the *BMJ*; being dreamers not doers we have thought of a name—the Clegg scholarship, after one of the journal's most distinguished editors—but haven't actually done anything to make it happen.)

The slings and arrows of an outrageous profession

En passant in his letter Dr Blum raises some important general points about a career in medical journalism or editing. He advises newcomers that both medical journals and medical editors are vulnerable, and, like any commercial organisation—but unlike the National Health Service—a medical journal (even one that is 150 years old), may disappear without warning. Dr Blum writes: "I see little if any hope for the continuation of full time physician editor positions in the US or Australia except as employees of drug companies." In this country medical publications have been hit hard by the government curtailing drug advertising, and several are likely to disappear. And editors are as easily wounded as their organs. Dr Blum writes: "A medical editor is an especially vulnerable role. Political and commercial considerations always seem to be just beneath the surface and can come up at any time. Each

The number of doctors working for various medical publications, what they do, how

Journal	Address	Full time doctors	Regular part time doctors	Number of expected vacancies for doctors in the next five years	How the do Writing and researching	Repo
British Medical Journal	BMA House, Tavistock Square, London WC1H 9JR	5	2	—	10	
Lancet	7 Adam Street, London WC2	3	hundreds	2		Very var
General Practitioner	76 Dean Street, London W1	1	1	Impossible to say	40	3
Medical News	359 Strand, London WC2	3	10	Possibly two	55	4
World Medicine	Surrey House, Throwley Way, Sutton, Surrey	—	1	—	5	
British Journal of Hospital Medicine	Northwood House, 93 Goswell Road, London EC1V 7QA	1	6	—	15	
The Practitioner	Calderwood Street, London SE18	1	2	One or two	5	1
Pulse	Calderwood Street, London SE18	1	1	Impossible to say		They c
Physician	Northwood House, 93 Goswell Road, London EC1V 7QA	1	1	Impossible to say	10	1

The editorial director of *Doctor* declined to answer our questions on the grounds that the information we asked for "v somewhat confidential nature." He added, "in the highly competitive field I feel it is inappropriate to comply wi request."

editor is an island, not only from journal to journal but within the sponsoring medical society."

But to set against these slightly gloomy thoughts and prognostications, there is a fun, if somewhat disreputable, side to medical journalism. Health matters occupy more and more space in the lay media, and doctor journalists are in demand. Even if your mornings and afternoons are occupied with the scholarly and ponderous, you can devote your dawns or nights to something more popular. Dr Blum spells out how this side of medical journalism is further advanced in the United States: "TV shlock docs are the latest thing in the US and are proliferating, adding the imprimatur of the MD news reader to the latest miracle cure, all sponsored by a vitamin or corn oil company. Indeed, this area of 'medical journalism' is about the only one that I am ever asked about. Everybody wants his own TV show, and the motives are strictly financial with a good dollop of plain vanity."

134

are paid, and what qualities the editors look for in applicants for the jobs

e their time (%)

cting ers	Subediting	Administration	Salary in comparison with NHS	Features particularly looked for in an applicant
o	15	10	Same	Wide clinical experience. Must be keen to pursue their own particular interests and ideas
t answer			Worse	—
o	5	5	Same	A few years general experience. Journalistic experience is an advantage but training can be given
5	o	o	Same	Must have a real commitment to journalism—this is not a way out for a doctor who is dissatisfied with clinical practice
st of the work is commissioning			Worse	—
o	30	20	Worse	Wide clinical experience is important as it gives the journalist some standing with his colleagues
o	35	20	Better	Must have—or be prepared to get—journalistic experience in order to make sense of the job
e things			Same	General practice experience and vocational training are essential. Journalistic training can be given through the company's training scheme
o	60	o	Same	Personality and outlook are important

So, in conclusion, the world of medical journalism is small, varied, and bitchy and is probably not for the faint hearted but may be an endless source of amusement to the thick skinned divergent thinker.

FOOTNOTE: Writing an article in tandem is always a difficult business, and reading it through afterwards one of us (SL) thinks that the other (RS) has called too many of the shots and made medical journalism and editing sound much more disreputable than they actually are. We therefore end by repeating Sarah Jenkin's important point that medical editing and journalism are not a refuge for the destitute doctor: you must want to be a journalist or an editor and have something to offer.

Appear on television

KARL SABBAGH

Why should a doctor need to know how to appear on television? Is an invitation to take part in a television programme so frequent that it is worth including in a book like this one? And, even if it is, is there anything the invitee can do himself that will contribute to the success or failure of the experience?

The answer is "yes" to both these questions. In the United Kingdom alone there are currently four television channels producing factual programmes, and cable television may bring more. The appetite for programmes in general and medical programmes in particular appears to be voracious, and the chances of some programme or other seeking your cooperation in a year are quite high. The invitation is even more likely to come if you are (a) involved in research, (b) active in medical politics, (c) a self publicist, or (d) negligent, incompetent, or criminal.

Since quite a high proportion of doctors come into one of those categories, so might you. In which case, it is only a matter of time before you pick up the phone to hear an imperious voice on the phone from Shepherds Bush or Charlotte Street inviting you to be filmed or recorded for a television programme. What, then, should be your reply, and how can you best make use of the opportunity?

If you pride yourself on being good with people, and many doctors do, then you should see the invitation as a useful test of your skills in this area. Television is run by people, after all, and if you can quickly establish a personal relationship with the people responsible for the television programme, you are more likely to be treated fairly and to be kept informed about what is going on. Terrorists and hostages provide a useful object lesson in this situation, since it seems that once any sort of good relationship is set up between terrorist and captor the hostage is probably safe. A superficial knowledge of or contempt for television can lead some doctors to keep their distance, try to exert their authority and

136

generally remain aloof even if they have agreed to cooperate in a programme. If they do that, I suggest, they are losing the opportunity to use the occasion effectively.

While it is easy to say "establish a good relationship with the television people", it is sometimes quite difficult to find out who they are. You may have a name or two as a result of that first phone conversation but it may be very difficult to find out exactly what role those names play in the production. There is an understandable tendency for each member of a television team to claim personal responsibility for both the idea and the work behind a programme. This is not always true. There are actually four main job descriptions you will come across—researcher, director, producer, and occasionally, executive producer. Each of these is involved in some way with production and each will persuade you that he holds the reins of power. If you know the functions of each of these you can actually use one against another to find out what you need to know about the programme to help you decide whether to appear at all.

The first person to call you is likely to be the researcher, trawling the professional world connected with the topic of the programme. Treat him or her politely, give an impression of great depth and originality, but don't waste too much breath, particularly if you are in the middle of a busy surgery or outpatients. Do, however, offer to send some printed material that describes your views or your work, and, unless you are dead set against any appearance on television for any reason at all, keep the channels of communication open.

The reason you are not spending too much time talking to the researcher is that he or she won't really be able to give you the answers to the important questions that you need to have answered before you can make your decision to help. These are: Who else will be appearing? Why was the topic chosen in the first place? Is it film or studio? Will it be edited afterwards? Will you be told how much of your contribution is finally to be used? Will any independent medical adviser see the programme before it goes out? And so on.

These questions can only really be answered by the producer, one or two rungs up the ladder. The researcher may give you answers, but you cannot hold him to them because he doesn't make the decisions. His research is passed on to the producer, or producer/director who is in charge of the programme, and who will have some control over the answers to the above questions.

One of the most puzzling distinctions to outsiders is the difference between the functions of a producer and a director in television. Confusion arises because, while production and direc-

137

tion are separate functions in a television programme, they are often performed by the same person.

A television programme usually starts with an idea by a producer who then writes a treatment, prepares a budget, gets together a team, and starts work. Decisions relating to staff, finance, and content are usually all his or hers. One member of his team could be the director of the programme. His or her job is to ensure that the pictures and sound that will be needed to tell the story arrive in a suitable form for transmission. If it is a film programme, this will involve planning to shoot the film, directing the film crew on location, and supervising the film editing in the cutting room. If it is a studio programme the director's role is concerned with the placing of cameras, the design of the set, and any subsequent editing of the videotape. In either of these media the director will be responsible to the producer. Any decision about your role in the programme, how the material is to be edited, the overall arguments to be presented—all of these are made or approved by the producer.

What sort of people are television producers, and what do you need to know about them and their job to make the most of your television opportunity? First of all, they are people who believe that television has a different role in society from the one many doctors think it should have. You must remember, if approached to appear on television, that broadcasting is not an arm of the public health services. One of its roles, and the one you are most likely to be consulted about, is to act as an honest reporter of the society we live in. So television producers are continually on the lookout for things which people do not know about and which, in their judgement as journalists, they think people would like to know about. In the health area this can range from new treatments to hospital closures, from drug disasters to prevention of heart disease. But a topic is rarely chosen because the producer feels that the viewers should know about it, for the good of their health. Unfortunately, since the good of the nation's health features largely in the priorities of many doctors, there is a source of conflict in the different approaches to publicising of health matters, which will exist until we have government—or BMA—controlled television.

But why is an appreciation of this conflict useful to a doctor who is invited to appear on television? Well, I believe that the best approach is a realistic one, and a doctor who has low expectations of what he will achieve on television will come away far more satisfied than one who sees it as a long sought chance to (a) publicise his life's research, (b) increase his grant, (c) improve the figures for his hypertension clinic, (d) get a dig in at his rivals.

138

If you are invited to appear on television your participation is likely to be in the form of an interview, unless you can juggle or do card tricks. Few programmes are transmitted live these days, so your contribution will probably be either filmed or recorded on videotape some time before it is transmitted as part of a programme. Although doctors are suspicious of recorded programmes because of the opportunities provided to the television production team for editing, I believe that prerecording allows a greater flexibility for participants as well as producers. I have known of producers who have spent hundreds of feet of valuable film filming several attempts by inexperienced interviewees to put over their points as well as possible.

Here are a few suggestions to help you make the most of an invitation to appear on television.

• Be limited in the amount you expect to get over. You are likely to be seen or heard for seconds rather than minutes, and if you cannot say something brief and useful about the topic of the programme, then don't accept the invitation. Bear in mind, however, that if you were asked to summarise your life's work by an acquaintance in some social setting, you would probably come up with quite a useful account, clear and comprehensible to a layman, in a couple of minutes.

• Accept the need for some editing of your contribution. After all, if you spoke to a newspaper reporter for ten minutes, you wouldn't expect him to print every word you said to him, 600 or so. You do have a right to be edited fairly, and you should certainly make it clear to the producer that you would like to be informed about what portion, if any, of your contribution remains in the final version of the programme. This is a courtesy you are entitled to, but is unlikely to be offered spontaneously to you. As well as giving you an opportunity to make a final plea for reconsideration if you don't like what the television people have done to you, it helps to avoid the embarrassing situation of your whole family sitting around to watch a programme from which you have unaccountably disappeared.

• Never address the camera—see it as an observer of the events of the programme, rather than as the focus for your remarks. Even if an interviewer is not seen in vision with you, there will usually be someone, the director or the researcher, to address your remarks to.

• If you are taking part in an interview or discussion don't be afraid to correct the interviewer or chairman, or to lead the discussion into areas that you would rather deal with. Many interviewees are too polite, and feel they must play according to the rules set by the television programme. This can lead to a situation where a participant saves up until after an interview something he should have pointed out during it.

I may have given the impression that, if you want to appear on television, you have to wait for someone to invite you. But increasingly, doctors themselves are suggesting opportunities for themselves or their colleagues, by building on contacts that they have made professionally or socially. No television producer minds receiving a well thought out programme suggestion from a viewer. What he does mind is receiving a suggestion for a programme which is identical to one transmitted in the last few weeks. If you feel there are things that television should be doing in your subject area, make sure first of all that these things aren't being done already, by watching television occasionally.

In fact, if there's one piece of advice I would offer above all others to someone invited to appear on television it is: to watch as much factual television as possible before you take part. Note what you find irritating or insincere or confusing or difficult to understand, and make a mental note to avoid those pitfalls yourself. You might even find the experience of watching television enjoyable in itself, and if you treat the medium seriously so will your viewers when you appear on it.

Prepare a lecture

R SHIELDS

Most of us receive an invitation to deliver a lecture with some pleasure. After all, it is an opportunity to speak at length, usually without interruption, to an audience of whom at least some wish to hear what we have to say. Unfortunately the audience may not share the pleasure. All too often the invitation is slipped into a drawer and little thought given to the lecture until a few days beforehand. The speaker who assumes that a carousel of hastily prepared slides and the mellifluence of his voice will see him through will leave the audience ill informed and dissatisfied, convinced that the hour devoted to the lecture could have been better spent. It is not trite to say that time spent preparing a lecture is never wasted.

The preparation of a lecture begins with the acceptance of the invitation. You must find out what your host expects and what the members of your audience are looking for—a description of your own research, a general review of recent advances, or a detailed description of practical procedures. What is the mix of the audience? Is there a predominant group with specific objectives—for example, to pass an examination? The most difficult and challenging lecture is without doubt one to a mixed audience, for example an inaugural lecture by a new professor to the staff of a large university, or a presidential lecture to a medical society when spouses and lay guests are present.

Title

Usually you will be asked to give a title when you accept the invitation so that the lecture can be widely advertised. The title should be informative, clearly defining the scope of the lecture. Avoid the vague, whimsical title, which conveys little or nothing to the potential audience. Try in the title to indicate your approach: whether didactic (for example, describing a procedure), provocative (reviewing current concepts and advances), or philosophical (viewing the topic in a much wider context than, for example, merely clinical). The title should be crisp, but not so brief that it does not indicate for whom the lecture is intended. In short, a title should have punch.

Content

In deciding what you are going to say, it is often valuable to define how your lecture would differ from a written communication for a medical journal. A lecture affords you certain opportunities. A lecture can be enhanced by the personality of the speaker, who by his enthusiasm can stimulate the audience. Difficult, or contentious, points can be repeated for emphasis, in a way that is not acceptable in a written communication. You can readily express opinions. You may speculate. You can present hypotheses which you would not wish to commit to paper. Results of unpublished or incomplete work can be described. These features can be contained within a lecture and may add to its enjoyment by providing a personal flavour. On the other hand, a written publication quite properly contains long descriptions of methodology and statistical analyses, complex tables, and graphs, all of which would be out of place in a lecture. Too much information should be avoided.

Prune the draft lecture ruthlessly. You are the expert, and your knowledge and experience are greater than most of the audience who can easily be lost or bored with minutiae. Try to limit yourself to one or two aspects of the subject and avoid an encyclopaedic coverage.

You will have to keep within a time limit. For most lectures an hour is set aside, but you should plan to speak for no more than 40–45 minutes.

At this stage you should discuss the scope and content of your lecture with a sympathetic colleague, preferably someone who could be a member of the audience. Try to find out what he, or she, would look for in the lecture: ask him, or her, to identify deficiencies in knowledge, so that you will know what to include to give your audience an elementary grasp of the subject.

Form

A lecture must be seen to possess a structure, so that the audience can more readily follow in the direction which you hope to lead them. Various formats are acceptable, but at the very least it should have: an introduction, the main body of the lecture, and a conclusion.

Introduction

The introduction has several uses. It enables the members of the audience to get to know you. They can become adjusted to your voice and hopefully to your manner. The introduction also allows you to become acquainted with the size and disposition of the audience in the room. You must try immediately to capture the audience's attention.

You should design your introduction to put forward several important points—the problem areas in the subject should be defined and the objectives which you are setting for yourself outlined. In preparing the introduction you should aim to stimulate the audience, prepare it for the main message, supply the basic information for an understanding of the subject, and establish a relationship with the audience.

There are many ways of introducing the lecture—by an historical allusion, by reference to previous speakers, by an anecdote, even by a provocative statement. You should aim for maximum impact. Occasionally with eponymous lectures, you are expected to allude to the person, or organisation, whom the lecture commemorates. This should always be done, but without obsequiousness or embarrassment to the audience. The link between the lecture and the person it commemorates should not be convoluted. For example, a link between John Hunter and monoclonal antibodies is not immediately apparent to most people: you should avoid too strained an allusion.

A successful introduction will leave the audience wishing, indeed demanding, to hear more.

The main body of the lecture

In preparing the body, or main message, of the lecture, there are several points that you should consider:

(1) Let the audience perceive the structure of the main part of your lecture. The format can be variable: for example, methods, results, conclusions; or review of published work, your own experience, discussion of your own results and those of others, and general applications. If you clearly demonstrate to the audience that there is order and structure to your lecture you can take them with you.

(2) It is in the middle part of a lecture that the skill and experience of a speaker become apparent. The audience, we

assume, has been attracted by the title and stimulated by the introduction. There is a risk, however, that about 20 minutes into the lecture its attention will begin to flag. The experienced lecturer, while keeping to his overall plan, should be prepared to vary the pace of his lecture at this point. Avoid proceeding too rapidly into the unfamiliar. You must prepare your lecture to allow yourself some flexibility, so that you can react with the audience—perhaps recapitulating facts previously mentioned, or recalling knowledge already familiar to the audience. Be prepared to break the direction and thrust of the lecture by an anecdote or provocative statement. It is important for the speaker to be aware of this mid-lecture dip in interest. You must not be too rigid or restricted in what you are going to say.

You should consider introducing a change in pace in the second half of the lecture; perhaps be more philosophical, perhaps retain the illustrations for this part of the lecture. You should lead your audience towards the crescendo which forms the conclusion of the lecture.

(3) You will have to decide whether or not to speak freely or read from a script. The introduction and conclusion should be carefully prepared, scripted and rehearsed; for the main body of the lecture, the structure and salient points only should be memorised. Usually it is better to speak freely. In this way you can look at the faces in the audience as you speak, and determine whether they are, as you hope, expectant and interested or, unhappily, bored and inattentive. With the printed paper in front of you, you may not respond to the audience. The read lecture can be enthralling, but considerable skill is required in its delivery. Much depends on the importance of the message and the personality of the speaker. The disadvantage of the read lecture is that the lecturer may speak monotonously into the lectern, giving the audience the impression that he does not wish to make any contact. The lecturer may be so bound to the printed page that he is afraid to free himself to move from the lectern to point out salient features of the slides. Sometimes even the speaker begins to sound bored with the lecture.

If you write out the entire text of the lecture to have it before you, you must appreciate the differences between the spoken and written words. In speaking words are simple and sentences short and of simple construction. If you wish to speak from a written script read it out several times to others, or into a taperecorder, and modify it until it flows as easily and naturally as the spoken word. Delivery of the written word requires considerable skill and rehearsal to ensure that pauses and changes of pace are included, and natural gestures introduced.

My advice is to speak, rather than read, a lecture. Notes or cards can be prepared as aides memoire. The text of these should be concise and brief as possible. You must be familiar with them, so that when you consult them there will not be an embarrassing pause while you try to decipher the writing, or reacquaint yourself with a new theme in your lecture. The typescript should be clear and written only on one side, each card clearly numbered. Thick wads of notes, or a sheaf of galley proofs, can be most off putting to the audience.

(4) Illustrations: speakers who graduate from the 10–15 minute paper to the 50 minute lecture may conclude that if 10 slides are appropriate for a short communication, 40–50 slides are necessary for a lecture. Slides, projected every minute in a darkened or semidarkened room will leave even the most interested audience asleep within 15 minutes. Good slides, the design and content of which are a task in themselves, should preferably be projected in sequences, so that the lights are not being continually switched on and off in a distracting manner during the lecture. Slides, videotapes and films may be kept to the latter half of the lecture, when the audience's interest may be flagging. Slides should not be used to jog the memory of the lecturer, but to emphasise the spoken word, to provide the audience with a visual memory, or perhaps, to show them in an illustration something which would take some time to describe in words. Unfortunately slides are often used by the nervous and insecure lecturer as a blanket to insulate himself from the audience.

There is, today, an increasing vogue for double projection. In expert hands, with, say, one slide displaying a concept and the other details, this technique can produce excellent results. Frequently it is just a device to swamp the audience with even more detail. The lecturer should not attempt double projection in a lecture room, or with equipment, with which he is not familiar.

Conclusion

You must clearly define the conclusion of your lecture, not just stop talking. The conclusion should be well prepared, rehearsed, and come over in a crisp, upbeat manner. Remember that the audience often feels pleased and satisfied if you return to concepts and ideas mentioned in the introduction. An audience likes to feel that, at least for the moment, the subject has been wrapped up. Do not include new facts or concepts in your conclusion. However you choose to conclude, the audience should be made aware that you are concluding: you should finish strongly, almost inviting the audience to break out into spontaneous applause.

Immediate preparations

You can very often allay the nervousness which you may feel, and increase your confidence that nothing will go wrong, by careful preparation immediately before giving the lecture. You must ask your host to let you see the lecture room beforehand. Look at the disposition of seats, whether you have to extend your neck to deliver your words to the back of highly tiered seats, or to throw them to the back of a flat room. Check the acoustics. Try, if possible, not to use a microphone but if you must, use one which is held around the neck rather than fixed, so that you can walk from the lectern to the screen. What is the lectern like? Some are simple; others with buttons, switches, and dials resemble the flight deck of Concorde. Become familiar with the essential switches. Make sure that you are not obscured by a large lectern—and be prepared to step aside from it, particularly during the introduction and conclusion. Look at the relative positions of the lectern and screen, for you must avoid running back and forward between them during the course of the lecture. Have a test slide projected to check that you can see it easily and not have to crane your neck to do so. Decide who will change the slides—yourself or a projectionist—and give the projectionist clear instructions about switching lights on and off. It is usually useful to have, as the first slide in the carousel, one which can be used exclusively for focusing and is unrelated to the rest of the lecture, so that you do not have to show the audience your first slide which is usually one with some impact. Look for pitfalls—a narrow platform, stairs, wires, stools that you may fall over or down. Check how to operate overhead projectors and videotape films. If you are going to use the blackboard, see that chalk and a duster are available. Check that there is a pointer and, if it is an electric one, determine how it works and particularly out of which end the light comes. Remind yourself to put the pointer down when not in use. There is nothing more distracting to an audience than to have the red spot of a laser beam dancing over the ceiling and the members of the audience.

Preparing oneself

Of all the preparations, perhaps the most difficult, is of yourself. Remember that a feeling of tension and nervousness is a frequent accompaniment of any major performance. Once you get into the body of the lecture and talking about a subject which interests you, your nervousness will go. Many accomplished lecturers would be concerned if they did not experience some tension beforehand.

146

We have enjoyed memorable lectures delivered by highly skilled and polished speakers. There are those who possess acting skills, and who, by gestures, pauses, and force of delivery, can capture and retain the attention of the audience. These skills are usually acquired by experience—by careful preparation and rehearsal, and by clear sighted analysis of each lecture after it has been given, to determine how it might be modified in the future.

A lecture is a bit of a performance, quite a challenging one because you have to write the script as well as deliver the lines. Remember that the members of the audience have usually come of their own accord and, at least initially, will be on your side. If you are speaking on a subject on which you have knowledge, and radiate your enthusiasm, if you show that you have given your lecture careful preparation and quickly establish a rapport with your audience, you will be successful in making the audience enjoy itself and receptive to the new concepts and information. The time spent in preparation will have made the lecture worthwhile both to yourself and to the audience.

Give a lecture

RICHARD LEECH

Speak the speech, I pray you.

Contrary to popular belief, the gifts of the actor, such as they are, are quite different to the gift of the gab. The trouble is that, although I have picked up a few wrinkles on making myself heard in public over the past forty years, I have previously had the benefit of cleverer and more articulate fellows to write the words. It's a different kettle of fish when you have to make it up yourself.

However, needs must when the devil and the Editor of the *BMJ* drive. I have lately done a bit of research and studied the form at a few centres of postgraduate learning. This is quite simple nowadays, for since the Minister has seen fit to award a bonus to GPs who attend such centres there has been a mushroom growth. There is hardly a hospital in the kingdom now which doesn't shove out the postgraduate boat—often loaded to the scuppers with goodies from the drug companies.

I have been amazed to discover how few of the lecturers at these establishments have bothered to consider the basic principles of voice production and presentation: principles without which no actor would ever achieve his first job. Thus I have been encouraged to believe that I have something to tell you that may be of help. I am not concerned with what you say. You have had expert advice on how to marshal your facts. I am only presuming to offer a few hints on how to say them.

First of all, then, you need to take up a position in good light where you can be comfortably seen by every member of the audience. An actor knows all about this. It is a truism to say that a selfish actor grabs the centre of the stage. But he does it for the very good reason that it is the easiest place from which to command an audience. As far as possible he will speak "out front" rather than "up stage" or "into the wings". If he can, he will avoid speaking on the move. These are not arbitrary fashions. They are immutable laws which he breaks at his peril.

148

In my researches I have discovered that many lecturers bury their heads in their notes, quickly narcotising their audience by having an intimate love affair with their own handwriting. With confidence born of thorough rehearsal, it should not be necessary to consult notes, unless the performer is using them as a device to enable him to draw aside and let a particular passage sink home. You remember Antony in his funeral oration:

"My heart is in the coffin there with Caesar,
And I must pause till it come back to me."

The actor who carries the book on stage with him is unlikely to win any awards, but for doctors, who after all have other more pressing calls on their time than the perfection of the actor's art, notes may be excused. But they must be used as memory aids and not read from. One topic ended, the lecturer should drop his head, read in silence, compose his new thoughts, then lift his head and continue his lecture.

There is a particular danger in case history notes. I came upon many doctors who were doing very nicely until they came to illustrating their point by reference to case notes. These notes record a particular triumph of diagnosis or treatment; otherwise the doctor wouldn't have bothered to bring them with him. But he has forgotten the details. That's why he needs the notes. As he refreshes his memory, he becomes fascinated by his own past brilliance, totally forgets his audience, and, with his nose deep in the notes, lapses into mumbling anecdotage.

Talking up stage

I am deaf and depend heavily on lip-reading, so I am particularly harassed by a performer who turns away. But even for people with the ears of an elk hound, lip reading plays a part, as does facial expression, and communication is restricted when the head is turned away. There are occasions when it is unavoidable—for example, drawing on a black-board or demonstrating the details on a slide. Actors call it "talking up stage," and when they can't escape it they make a particular effort to lift their voice and project more clearly in order to overcome it.

The pointer is another hazard which encourages the exhibition of the Dick Whittington syndrome. This is where the lecturer shoulders his pointer and sets out on the last ten miles for London, becoming so engrossed in his route march that he loses his audience by the way. Many postgraduate centres are now equipped with microphones, but unless you are lecturing in a football field it is possible to do without them. Indeed, for all but experts they are apt to do more harm than good. The major danger, I think, is the temptation to use the microphone as a charm which will ward off evil and magically transform an unconfident, ill-prepared mumbling attack of verbal diarrhoea into an interesting and audible discourse. I have seen—I can't say heard—many performers groaning away, making not even the natural effort they would to speak across a room, in the complacent belief that the microphone is transforming all. If you use a microphone you have to speak into it from a distance which remains nearly constant. Rapid variation in the distance causes electronic thunderstorms. This problem can be overcome by a chest mike—which should be hung six to nine inches from the mouth. I sat under a London consultant lately who inherited the chest mike from a Scottish giant, and failed to adjust the neck strap. The instrument hung like a string of bones round a witch doctor's neck. It may have worked like a charm for him, but it didn't help us, and after a while we even gave up listening to the borborygmi. The chest mike can add a complication to the Dick Whittington syndrome if you allow the lead to get tangled up with your legs.

Breath the creator

In the beginning was the word. But in order to transmit it you need breath. Breath is the great creator. God breathed on a handful of dust to create man. It is impossible to exaggerate the importance of filling the lungs with air. A chestful of air is a wonderful antidote to butterflies in the stomach. That ghastly moment when you stand surveying the many-headed monster, courage oozing from the heels of your shoes, can be converted to a moment of confidence if you stop worrying and concentrate on taking a really deep breath.

Good breathing automatically neutralises a whole catalogue of faults—for example, the infuriating lack of communication which results from dropping the ends of sentences. This is caused by a dwindling in the supply of air in the lungs, until there is no longer enough to carry the sound away and so it drowns in a gurgle in the throat. Actors use this shortage of breath to effect. We call it "throwing away a line," and lots of consultants I heard are on to it. It can be a witty sophisticated effect. But, as Nöel Coward said, if you're throwing a line away, you need to be quite sure where you are throwing it. Though it should come across as an aside—an afterthought or snide comment on your own lecture—it is, of course, totally valueless unless it is heard.

In a brief tip-sheet of the most obvious faults of voice production, I have only space for one more. It is the question of where you "place" your voice, how you use—or fail to use—the resonant cavities of your head. Some lucky people place their voices naturally forward in the front of the mouth and their words wing happily to their audience. But others keep the sound trapped in the back of their throat, a fault exaggerated by the tightened muscles of nervousness. It is a particularly English complaint. Celts tend not to be so afflicted. In extreme cases you get the state of affairs celebrated in the story about the New York barman who said to his visitor, "Say—you're English aren't ya?" and the stranger replied, "If I were any more English I couldn't talk at all."

It is a fault more difficult to eradicate than most others. Sufferers tend not to be able to distinguish the difference in placing. Once you can hear the difference, you can't bear to make the mistake. Chronic sufferers really need expert advice, but a brief first aid treatment which has helped me is to repeat, "Teeth—lips—tip of the tongue—" over and over, at the same time trying to feel the resonance in your antra and the front of your face.

Use Slides

MARY EVANS

"What is conceived well is expressed clearly"—BOILEAU

The standard of verbal delivery of scientific lectures has improved in recent years (largely as a result of the insistence of research societies that papers must not be "read") but that of visual presentation has lagged behind. Audiences are expected to tolerate bad slides, despite the efforts of such pioneers as Hawkins,[1] Calnan and Barabas,[2] and Dudley.[3]

"None can be said to know things well who do not know them in their beginnings"[4]; perhaps lack of understanding of the three purposes of slides (background, evidence, and illustration) is at the root of their continuing mediocrity. They should be used to put the work in perspective, to give a distillation of the evidence for the case being presented, and to illustrate the results.

They must not be used as aides mémoire. Poor speakers who face the screen and declaim the text of each slide to the last syllable do nothing but irritate their audience. The correct function of slides is to complement a talk in the same way that pictures enhance an advertisement and "give a truthful, exact, apt and striking description of the goods advertised."[5]

Many lessons may be learned from the world of advertising. Ogilvy[5] wrote that "The purpose of illustration is to telegraph the message the reader" and a useful rule is that if a slide cannot be understood by the audience in four seconds it is a bad slide; if people have to concentrate on working out the message of a slide they are not listening to the speaker. Good slides can be shown at the rate of one every 50 seconds.

There are seven adjectives which describe good slides: appropriate, accurate, legible, comprehensible, well executed, interesting and memorable. If any of these cannot be used to describe your slides, scrap them and start again.

152

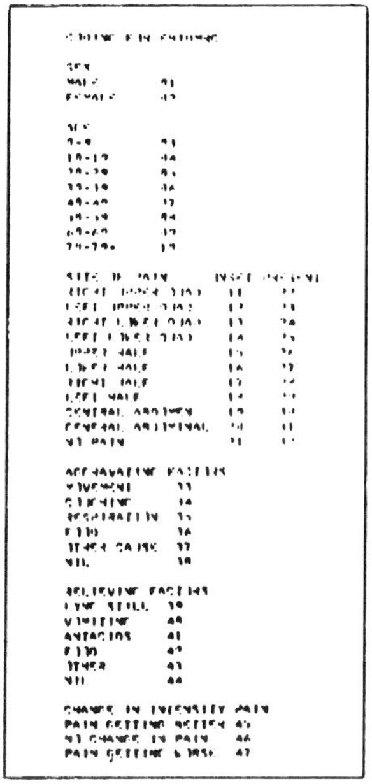

Fig 1—*Inappropriate. A computer print-out has been photographed. The proportions are wrong, there is far too much on the slide, and contrast is poor.*

Appropriate

Tables, graphs, and drawings produced in enough detail for journals (where they may be studied at leisure) are unsuitable for slides (fig 1). The salient points should be abstracted and, where possible, presented as pictures, cartoons, or diagrams that produce an immediate effect. If words must be used, then only a précis should be given. Yorke[6] showed the virtue of abbreviation when he pointed out that if Nelson's signal had read "With reference to previous instructions appertaining to naval discipline, it is felt that all personnel in the immediate vicinity of Cape Trafalgar will carry out the navigational and/or combative duties allocated to them, whichever is applicable, to the satisfaction of all concerned" instead of "England expects that every man will do his duty," it would have been neither obeyed nor remembered.

Accurate

"I do not mind lying but I hate inaccuracy"—SAMUEL BUTLER

It should be unnecessary to make this point. I have, however, seen the following spelling mistakes on slides shown recently at

153

national and international meetings: ileostemy, strep pneumonae, anticoagulent, femero-femoral, ilio-rectal, intermittant and—one of the most common—anastamosis.

Richard Asher's[7] plea is well-founded—"However good your memory is, you should look up everything you quote." One should add "and then check it again." This is particularly true if the slides are being typed by someone lacking a detailed knowledge of technical terms. Always check the artwork for spelling before having it photographed.

Errors are not always accidental, nor are they restricted to text. When drawing a graph, for example, it is possible to show bias to the point of dishonesty if you draw it with a vertical axis showing 40% at the bottom and 45% at the top, instead of 0 and 100% (fig 2).

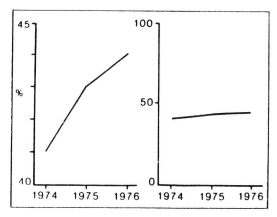

Fig 2—*Inaccurate. These two graphs give the same information but the one on the left is misleading.*

Legible

The size of a slide is 35×22 mm. Whatever you are showing—text, diagram, pie chart, histogram, graph—the proportions of 35 to 22 should be strictly adhered to. Thus if the width is fixed you should multiply by 22 and divide by 35 to give the correct depth and, if the depth is fixed, you should multiply by 35 and divide by 22 to give the correct width. This ensures that full use is made of the space available. It is of vital importance that only a limited amount of information should appear on each slide, and this objective can be achieved by insisting that the presenter of the paper shall do his own artwork (fig 3). He will find that it takes

154

VERTEBRAL CANAL MEASUREMENTS (MM)

No.	Patient No.	Lumbar Vertebral Level	Anteroposterior		Interpeduncular	
			Scan	Caliper	Scan	Caliper
1	1	2	16	16	24	24
2		3	20	17	26	22
3	2	2	18	17	26	22
4		3	18	17	22	22
5	3	2	22	19	26	26
6		3	19	18	27	26
7	4	2	17	16	23	22
8		3	20	16	20	22
9	5	1	20	19	26	24
10		2	20	20	28	26
11		3	21	18	78	26
12		4	18	16	28	26
13	6	1	20	20	22	20
14		2	17	17	22	21
15		3	17	16	21	21
16		4	17	17	23	22
17	7	1	19	19	27	26
18		2	18	19	24	26
19		3	21	21	26	20
20		4	22	23	28	29
21	8	1	19	20	21	21
22		2	18	18	21	21
23		3	18	18	23	23
24		4	19	17	26	23

Fig 3—*Illegible and uninteresting. "Portrait" style. Too much information, dull, and means nothing.*

much less time to construct a simple slide. Medical art departments should concentrate on medical art, whether in drawings or photographs. Too often they are expected to produce sensible slides from material suitable only for publication. There is no better way for a speaker to clarify his thoughts than to be obliged to construct the slides himself.

Expensive equipment such as a Varafont (known in the United States as a Kroy), or Letraset, can help not only to make legible slides, but also to give them a professional appearance. Letraset (transfer lettering) is supplied in sheets. It produces excellent work when spacing and alignment are carefully measured, but the process is slow and expensive.

The Varafont (manufactured by Kroy Industries Inc, Stillwater, Minnesota, USA, and distributed in the UK by Murographics Ltd, Oldmixon Industrial Estate, Weston super Mare, Avon) prints from interchangeable fonts on to adhesive polyester acetate or paper tape with peel off backing. The tape is positioned on and stuck to a surface suitable for photography. With either method the optimum is 24 point type on A4 (297 × 210 mm) matt cartridge paper with margins of 30 mm all round. It should be possible to read the original artwork from a distance of four metres.

Though not nearly so attractive, it is quicker and cheaper to have the artwork typewritten. Type is measured in points, one point being 0·0138 of an inch. Most typewriters have letters which are either eight, 10, or 12 point and, if a slide is typewritten, the entire text must be confined to the space left on a postcard (140 × 90 mm) after you have ruled a 20 mm border at the top and bottom and a 30 mm border at each side. For tables Calnan and Barabas[2] suggest a maximum of four columns and seven lines but even this amount—if badly set out—cannot be read easily.

Make sure that the typewriter has no idiosyncrasies such as letters which are out of line or crooked. The keys (or daisy wheel) must be clean and not cracked; such defects are embarrassingly obvious on the screen. A carbon ribbon should be used, lines of lettering should be double spaced, and words separated by two letter spaces. Electronic typewriters which centre automatically have taken a lot of the drudgery out of setting out typewritten slides.

Many microcomputers are capable of displaying histograms and other figures on their visual display units (and of printing them in dot matrix form). As a rule these are not suitable for slides, which look better if the artwork is drawn with a black felt tipped pen.

Several other rules should be observed to achieve legibility. Firstly, never use full stops—they disturb the visual flow of type—and use other punctuation marks sparingly. Secondly, choose capital letters and lower case consistently (fig 4). Use capital letters for titles and lower case for text; it is more pleasing to see a line completely in upper case or completely in lower case, except where initial capitals must be used for proper names. People read lower case typescript more quickly and easily than upper case. Eric Partridge[8] quotes from the preface to Webster's International Dictionary of 1934: "It should be clear to even the meanest intelligence that the unnecessary use of capitals may easily lead to ambiguity or, at the least, to discomfort and resentment."

156

PLAIN RADIOLOGY - 50 PATIENTS

8 "Spinal Stenosis" Cases proved at Surgery

Measurement and "Ration Analysis" failed to isolate Stenosis Cases

Fig 4—*Ill-executed and inaccurate. Proportions wrong, capital letters scattered throughout, "ratio" misspelt and spacing inconsistent.*

Thirdly, use space between letters, words, and lines with care. In road signs the largest observed effect on reading distance is produced by changes in spacing.[9]

Fourthly, use a sans serif typeface (one without the "tails" on the letters). It is easier to read at a glance,[5] though a serif face is preferable on the printed page. Attractive and legible typefaces are Helvetica, Microgramma, and Univers.

Finally, in a "summary" slide asterisks or dots are more arresting than labelling points with figures, 1, 2, 3, etc. Quite apart from the visual effect, figures indicate a diminishing order of importance which is not always what one wishes to convey.

Comprehensible

How often have you heard a speaker comment apologetically "This slide may look rather complicated." It is usually an understatement and signifies only that he has not taken the time and trouble to simplify it. Complicated formulae and detailed experimental methods have no place on slides (fig 5). They need only be mentioned by the speaker, and those who want the details can be referred to published work.

Abbreviations, though tempting, should be used with care— particularly if the audience is international. Certain standard ones have been published,[10] but it is sensible to explain any others that you use.

$$var(S) = \frac{1}{18}\left\{n(n-1)(2n+5) - \sum_t t(t-1)(2t+5) - \sum_u u(u-1)(2u+5)\right\}$$
$$+ \frac{1}{9n(n-1)(n-2)}\left\{\sum_t t(t-1)(t-2)\right\}\left\{\sum_u u(u-1)(u-2)\right\}$$
$$+ \frac{1}{2n(n-1)}\left\{\sum_t t(t-1)\right\}\left\{\sum_u u(u-1)\right\}.$$

Fig 5—*Incomprehensible. Kendall's "S" statistic. Suitable for publication but not for a slide.*

Well executed

Though this is closely related to "legible," it should be remembered that "an ugly layout suggests an ugly product."[5] Slides should be well balanced and, where possible, designed to be shown horizontally (landscape) rather than vertically (portrait) as there are surprisingly few lecture halls in which the screen does not cut off one end of a vertical slide. Always write horizontally when annotating the vertical axis of a graph. Never, under any circumstances, do your final drawing on graph paper as the lines will confuse and distract (fig 6).

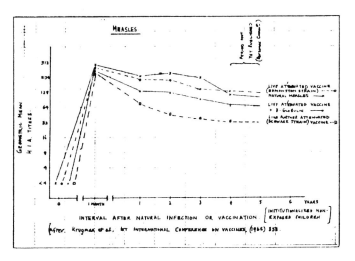

Fig 6—*Ill-executed. Too much information, badly drawn on graph paper, vertical lettering on the ordinate, etc.*

The choice of the method of photographic reproduction to use (colour, black on white, diazo or negative) is a matter of taste and opportunity. Dudley[3] states a preference for diazo as he finds the blue and white restful; some would describe it as soporific. Large traffic signs (such as directions on motorways) employ light coloured lettering on a dark background,[11] and this principle is applied both in diazo and negative slides.

The latter are the quickest and easiest for the amateur to produce, and colour can help to achieve balance as well as being important in other respects. It can be helpful to have all the headings or references to a particular feature in the same colour, and certain colours have natural associations which can be used to

158

advantage. We are brought up to recognise, for example, that red implies heat or danger, green safety, and blue peace or cold. A most useful colour is white, not only in its own right[12] but also to "point" or balance other colours.

If you are making your own negative slides you will need a single lens reflex camera, "Kodalith" 35 mm film, and the appropriate developers, two No. 2 Photofloods and—if your originals are typewritten—a No. 2 close up lens. The exposure is $\frac{1}{2}$ sec at f8. Colouring and mounting should be done at the same time and require back lighting, most simply provided by a portable x-ray screen. Slides need protection and should be mounted between glass; the grey and white Gepe mounts are ideal. Mount the transparency on the grey side, and secure it with masking tape. Then apply the colours directly to the face of the film, ideally using Staedtler Lumocolor pens (designed for use with overhead projectors). If you cannot get these any coloured felt tipped pen will do (for example, Golden Platignum "painting sticks"), though care should be taken as sometimes the points are rather thick. Any small flaws in the developing process (which show up as white dots or lines) can be concealed by using a black felt-tipped pen or masking tape.

Whichever type of production you choose, you will make a bad impression if your slides are not mounted straight or if they are dirty. Always put an adhesive dot in the bottom left hand corner of the mount to help the projectionist (there are seven incorrect ways of showing a slide). Check your slides just before handing them in; transparencies can slip within the mounts in transit, even when secured by tape. Take spare mounts with you, in case you find the glass of a vital slide broken.

Interesting

"You cannot bore people into buying."[5] If your slides are dull, inaccurate, badly made, and illegible your audience will either go to sleep or leave the hall. As Hopkins[13] pointed out, "A person who desires to make an impression must stand out in some way from the masses" and this is particularly important if you are presenting one of 50 or more papers at a research meeting where each one of your audience has his own axe to grind.

Memorable

There are few memorable slides. We all know which they are—we remember them.

Conclusion

I wish I could say with conviction (pace Samuel Johnson) that when a man knows he is to speak in a fortnight it concentrates his mind wonderfully. Even more do I wish that this would be reflected in the quality of his slides.

[1] Hawkins C. *Speaking and writing in medicine*. Springfield: Thomas, 1967.
[2] Calnan, J, and Barabas, A. *Speaking at medical meetings*. London: Heinemann Medical Books, 1972.
[3] Dudley, H A F. *The presentation of original work in medicine and biology*. Edinburgh: Churchill Livingstone, 1977.
[4] Temple, Sir William. Preface to History of England. Quoted by: St Arnaud, G. *Legislative power of England*. London: Thomas Woodward, 1725.
[5] Ogilvy, D. *Confessions of an advertising man*. London: Longmans Green, 1964.
[6] Yorke, G C. *Working with words*. London: Blackie, 1965.
[7] Asher, R. *Richard Asher talking sense*. London: Pitman Medical, 1972.
[8] Partridge, E. *The gentle art of lexicography*. London: Andre Deutsch, 1963.
[9] Christie, A W, and Rutley, K S. Relative effectiveness of some letter types designed for use on road traffic signs. *Roads and Road Construction* 1961; **39**: 239–44.
[10] International Steering Committee of Medical Editors. Uniform requirements for manuscripts submitted to biomedical journals. *Br Med J* 1979; i: 532–5.
[11] Moore, R L, and Christie, A W. *Research on traffic signs*. Proceedings of Conference of Engineering for Traffic. London: Printer Hall, 1963.
[12] Chesterton, G K. A piece of chalk. In: *Tremendous trifles*. Beaconsfield: Darwin Finlayson, 1968.
[13] Hopkins, C. *Scientific advertising*. London: McGibbon and Kee, 1968.

Use an overhead projector

T S MURRAY

An overhead projector is now a standard piece of equipment in most teaching departments. It is a most useful visual aid and can be used efficiently if a number of basic ground rules are followed.

During a lecture the overhead projector may be used to replace or supplement the blackboard. It is clean, provides the teacher with an almost limitless area, and allows him to face his audience. The room does not need to be darkened and the flow of presentation is therefore uninterrupted. The lecturer is responsible for his own transparencies and can control the order and timing of the material. He can also add to or alter the material during presentation.

A large surface area is provided by the acetate roll on the projector, which provides 50 feet of blackboard. The best results on the acetate roll are obtained by using a technical pen with special ink that can be either water soluble or permanent. When the page of acetate has been filled, the roll is wound on to reveal a clean surface. Later, if required, the roll can be wound back and used to recap on the session.

The screen should be mounted as high as possible so that the audience has a clear view. There are two common positions for the projector—either in the centre with the screen directly facing the audience, or with the screen placed obliquely in a corner with the projector in a corresponding position. On a vertical screen a tilted beam of light produces an image that is wider at the top than the bottom (keystone distortion). This effect is prevented by tilting the upper edge of the screen forwards.

Preparation of transparencies

Transparencies can be prepared at short notice (when the production of slides would be impossible)—an undoubted advantage when prepararation time is limited. Many doctors do not have access to audiovisual departments for producing slides, but can prepare transparencies themselves with minimal materials and reach an acceptable standard if care is taken in preparation.

If the transparencies are to form part of a permanent teaching package it is best to buy a box of acetate sheets. Cellofilm, which is cheaper, can also be used but it is flimsy and tends to curl when exposed to heat and moisture; x-ray film which has been developed can also be used, the simplest method of cleaning being to leave the sheets soaking in soap and water overnight. If none of these materials is available, polyethylene may be used.

When using acetate sheets it is necessary to use special pens, which can have either a spirit base or a water base. The advantage of the water based pens are that the acetate sheets can be washed and used again, an undoubted advantage when the material is used on only one occasion—for example, a case presentation. The pens are of various thicknesses, but all are easy to use. Special pens can be obtained at a graphics shop and these produce professional looking transparencies: stencils have also been produced to use with them. Ordinary pens are unsuitable on acetate but can be used on cellofilm. Normal typewriter type is too small to produce a satisfactory visual image for transparencies. Even if the height of the letter is increased, type which is 10–12 characters to the inch will appear too crowded. The solution centres on increasing the size of the projected image and typewriters are now available which are modified to provide a large character, at a frequency of around six to the inch. Golf ball typewriters with special heads can produce the large character.

The transparencies are mounted in cardboard, thus aiding storage and preventing damage. The mounts must not interfere with the visual content and at least 15 mm should be left between the inside of the frame and the outer limit of the content. Mounts also aid handling during presentation, and the registration pegs on the projector allow adequate positioning.

The most important aspect of any visual aid is communication with the audience and the material must be easily understood and legible. A blurred picture can be the result of dust on the lens and mirror but a poor transparency is a more likely cause. The whole of the transparency must be in focus. The transparencies may be used to introduce, illustrate, or consolidate a lecture. They can reinforce the important headings. Information must be restricted to eight words to a line and eight lines to a transparency. Use of several different colours can add to the impact of the transparency. Letraset produce self adhesive transfer letters if you are unhappy about printing, and self adhesive material in roll form. Letrafilm is a self adhesive colour film and this helps to emphasise points and give variety. Anatomical drawings can be traced directly on to acetates by using an episcope, which can reduce or enlarge the size of the drawing by projecting the image. If this equipment is not available, the drawing may be enlarged using the overhead projector itself. Trace the drawing by using cellofilm, project, and then trace directly on to acetate. Commercially available kits—for example, Letravision—are now available and allow a professional transparency to be prepared easily and quickly. The kits are accompanied by explicit instructions.

Specific techniques

Masking is used for uncovering information at various stages in a lecture. By using an ordinary sheet of plain white paper the lecturer can mask the whole transparency and reclaim the full attention of the class. By moving the paper, he reveals the teaching points one by one. He can read the text through the paper, and is thus in complete control of the presentation and can lead the discussion to a particular point before projecting the next line of notes. Use of the switch can also attract the audience's attention: switch off when you want the attention and switch on when the attention has to be given to the overhead.

A pen may point out on the transparency a specific part, word, or sentence to emphasise something that the lecturer thinks is important. But he must not wave the pen about, as this can be distracting. The pen can also be used to underline the point.

Silhouetting can be produced by laying objects on the stage and this often leads to better understanding—for example, of the position of a prosthetic valve during a lecture on cardiac surgery. Perspex models may also be used to illustrate difficult teaching points—for example, the actions of the intrinsic muscles of the larynx.

Overlays are a simple technique for adding to the versatility of the overhead projector. An overlay is a separate sheet which carries additional information and which is added to the main drawing or diagram. It is usually hinged down one side with adhesive tape and when required is turned over to lie flat on the stage—blood vessels, for example, can be placed over a diagram of a limb, and this could be followed by the peripheral nerve supply. Several different commercially prepared transparencies are now available in all medical subjects and the overlay technique allows you to explain complex diagrams.

The illusion of movement—blood flow, for example—can be achieved by using a special attachment which fits over the

163

projector's working surface. This calls for special materials and relies on the movement of one transparent film relative to another.

Many radiographs can be projected successfully with an overhead projector. For this purpose, the room has to be darkened and as much of the radiograph as possible masked off, so that there are no bright patches of light beyond the area of interest.

The overhead projector is a valuable, versatile visual aid—usually for lectures, but also for small groups. It can be used in a well lit room with the lecturer facing his audience and completely controlling his presentation. It can also be used to focus discussion in small group teaching, or to provide information with results in a group problem-solving exercise. It is a useful substitute for the blackboard, but with proper use is much more versatile.

Further reading

McRae, R K. *The Overhead projector*, Medical Education Booklet No. 4, Association for the Study of Medical Education, Dundee, 1975.

Construct an audiovisual programme

ELIZABETH A BRAIN, CHARLES M BIDWELL

Audiovisual technology provides powerful and varied methods of communication. Events and ideas may be presented as they happen to a large and widely distributed audience through such media as radio, telephone, and public or closed circuit television. Alternatively, by recording events and ideas on audiotape, slides, film, videotape, or videodisc such information may be presented at a later time and in a place convenient to the viewer or listener. Furthermore, recordings may be edited to suit specific educational objectives, or may be linked with a computer to provide randomly accessed illustrations for interactive and individualised instruction.

The medium and the message

The medium and the message are closely interrelated or, as Marshall McLuhan said, "The medium is the message." This interrelationship makes it difficult to decide which to consider first, and indeed you should consider the message and the medium in tandem. The message should influence the choice of medium; the medium should enhance the message. Too often, however, the medium shapes the message and can easily limit or distort it. The important factors that should influence both your choice of medium and the message are: your educational goals and objectives, your facilities and budget for production, and your facilities and budget for distribution, especially the equipment available to the user.

The message

As the author of an audiovisual programme you are the subject expert. You should therefore take pains to formulate your message accurately. Audiovisual technology has the power either to enhance or distort your message, but no audiovisual technique can create it. The form of the message will depend upon your subject and your audience and together these will determine your objectives. What is the nature of your topic? Will you be illustrating concepts, demonstrating a technique, or exemplifying interactions between individuals? Will you be addressing students, the lay public, or a group of practising health professionals? What is the quality and the quantity of learning that you wish them to achieve? What prerequisite knowledge must they have? How will your approach differ for each group, to facilitate the learning that you wish them to achieve?

The choice of medium

The objectives should guide your choice of medium. Unless the medium has been dictated to you by your producer, you should ask yourself these questions (see fig 1). What is necessary to achieve your educational objectives? Are visuals required? Should they be coloured? Is movement essential? Should the visuals be projected, or may they be printed? Is sound essential, or can the message be

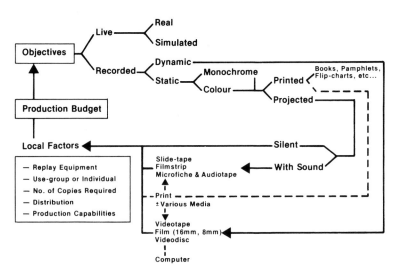

Fig 1—*A media decision tree—illustrates the factors which must be considered in deciding on an appropriate medium.*

166

conveyed with visuals or text alone? What local factors will affect your means of distribution? Finally, what budget will your plans require, and if there are financial limitations how must you modify your decisions to accommodate them? In addition, you may want to decide whether or not to combine the media with a study guide, a text, or a computer program. Whatever medium or combination of media you decide to use, there will be basic elements to your programme: the script, the visual display, the audio track, textual portion, and the complete package.

The script

It is essential to prepare a script which accurately sets out your message, bearing in mind that it will be illustrated and recorded. The script for an audiovisual programme grows and changes and does not become final until the production is completed. Nevertheless, you must commit your message to paper early on, so that it is your message which dictates the production and not the reverse. Aim at making a 15–20 minute programme unless otherwise specified. Remember you are not writing a paper: you will be heard, not read. Imagine you are talking to an individual or a small group. To achieve a spoken approach it helps to dictate your initial script. You should be direct, positive, active not passive, and conversational. Have your script typed on the right half of the page using double spacing, starting a new paragraph for each new idea or step, and leaving additional space between paragraphs for inserting editorial changes. The other half of the page should be used for notes about the visuals and other technical instructions. Try to think visually and plan your scenarios, illustrations, diagrams, or models in relation to your script, but if you cannot visualise a relevant illustration at this stage, do not panic, but proceed with your script logically. If you are writing for television or film, your script must be sufficiently detailed for the production crew to know what will be taking place, how long the narrative lasts for a specific camera view, and the importance of particular actions or manoeuvres so that they can follow the action and make close-up recordings appropriately. It is not, however, essential to provide full details of dialogue.

You will no doubt revise or edit your draft script, possibly after having it reviewed by colleagues or representatives of the intended audience, to clarify the message, rectify grammatical faults (often introduced in dictation), and later to respond to changes as they occur in production. Care in the preparation of your script should ensure the accuracy of your message.

The visual display

In any audiovisual programme, the visuals tend to be the primary stimulus, and should therefore make an impact. If you are using slides, you should have a new slide for each point; two to four slide changes a minute are not too many. Keep the slides simple, lucid, and varied. Colour should be used for emphasis and to coordinate related material, but should not be distracting. The visual style should be consistent and care should be taken to make certain that the sequence and juxtaposition of slides is appropriate. Try to establish a visual model which can be repeated or added to throughout the programme. Key words and technical and unfamiliar terms should be emphasised visually. Ensure that the narrative is relevant to the illustrations; a picture which is retained for too long rapidly loses impact.

You can use several slides to focus on different parts of a diagram and thus avoid having too many details on the screen at once. Complicated schemes, charts or diagrams may be built up sequentially by using overlays on a basic drawing. Changing visuals frequently will prevent you from presenting too much detail in each one. Graphs or tables used in textbooks or journals often contain too much information, and should be simplified for audiovisual programmes. Find a key word or a heading to use if a part of your narrative does not seem to be usefully illustrated by a graphic visual. Blank or solid colour slides are distracting or dazzling and should not be used, except to achieve a specific effect. Eliminate as much verbiage as possible from the visuals. Sentences need not be complete, key words alone may best make the point. A screen should display not more than eight lines of writing with a total of 15 to 20 words, and space at least the height of a capital letter between lines. Lower case script is usually easier to read than upper case script, though capital letters, as well as colour, may be used for emphasis. Cartoons and humour may be motivating and entertaining if, like perfume, they are used with discretion. Cartoons make a forceful impression, and so make certain that they impress the message you want remembered.

Many of the same principles apply when thinking about visuals for television. Remember that all still visuals intended for use in a video recording must be in horizontal and TV format—that is they must fit a ratio of $1:1.5$ in a framework of $2:3$ to be clearly visible on a television screen. The script for a camera recording of an event or personal interaction should identify the person who should be the centre of focus, whether the audience should see the interaction between two or more individuals, or the response of one, and from which angle. Always record sequences that are long

168

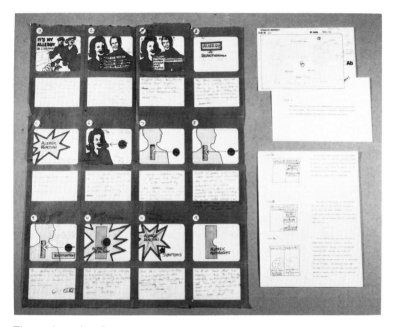

Fig 2—*A storyboard.*

enough to allow for editing, but not so long that you have to watch hours of videotape in order to select the scenes you want. This process takes time, and time is money!

Careful planning and matching of the text and visuals on paper is called a *storyboard*. Storyboards may take several forms, varying from one produced on specially prepared paper, to a series of cards each displaying either a visual or its matching text, to little more than an annotated script (see fig 2). The importance of a storyboard is threefold. Firstly, it enables you to balance the visuals and text and see that the message is conveyed correctly. Secondly, your draft programme may be shown to colleagues or students for their opinions before any major production has started. You may find it helpful to read your script while your colleague follows the visuals. Thirdly, it enables the artist to understand the points you are making and thus to execute the illustrations accurately.

The audio track

The audio portion of an audiovisual programme is where you can least afford to cut corners. Students will excuse homemade slides if they are relevant, but if they have to strain to hear what you are saying, are distracted by extraneous noise, are bored by a slow delivery, or cannot understand because of an accent, you will soon lose their attention. For this reason, many people feel that a professional narrator should be used, but, although professionals will provide a smooth sound track, they often lack conviction, tend to sound aloof, and mispronounce medical and scientific terms. Provided that you do not have a heavy accent, a speech impediment, or a monotonous voice, you should record the narration yourself because you can impart enthusiasm for your subject, and emphasise and pronounce certain words in a way that a professional cannot. If you are doubtful about your abilities, make a trial tape, and if necessary enlist the help of a colleague to narrate for you.

To ensure the best quality audio recording, try to use the services of an audio technician who will attend to the technical details, such as the position of microphones and the voice levels, and who can edit out coughs, page noises, unnecessary pauses, and so on. Master audio recordings should be made on reel to reel tape for the best quality and easy editing. Audiocassette tapes for distribution may be reproduced from these masters. You should make your audiotape by reading from the final script, which has been checked with the finished illustrations. If you originally dictated your script you will have a natural sounding narrative. Use a conversational manner, sound interested, and even excited; your students cannot see you; they have to hear your enthusiasm. Pace is important. Allow time for students to absorb the information. If you wish them to study a visual without further narration tell them. Students more often complain that tapes are too slow than too fast. They can stop and replay a tape, but they cannot speed up the narration.

Audiotapes should be checked with the slides after recording and before duplicating. It is preferable to add any slide change signals (audible or electronic) at this point, when the exact timing can be assessed.

The audio track of a videotape is laid down in several ways. It may be recorded simultaneously with the visual scene, or it may be produced first, carefully timed and the visuals added subsequently, or you may use "voice over" when you describe the visuals after the event. Most of the principles described for audiotapes apply to video as well, but you should discuss the method of approach with your producer.

A short musical introduction over titles and credits allows time for the student to settle down, to adjust the volume, and to focus the visual images on the screen. Beware of copyright, and try to use music which is in the public domain. Music may set the mood, but familiar melodies can also distract the listener's attention from the message, and recall unintended associations.

Text

Many audiovisual programmes have an accompanying handbook which enhances their educational value and flexibility. It is difficult to scan an audiovisual resource as one can a book, and so it is helpful to have certain information available in printed form. The text may contain such items as the educational objectives, a content outline, cataloguing information, including a summary, target audience and audience level, as well as technical information.

A transcript of the audiotape may be printed for preview, review, or as an alternative to the audiotape. References, test questions and answers, problems for practice, and detailed diagrams or tables, which may be too complicated for a visual but which require further study, may also be included in the text. If a handbook or study guide is not practical for your purpose, some of this key information should be supplied on the label of the container holding the programme.

The package

When you have completed the components, assemble them into a package. Slides should be numbered, and boxes and texts labelled. Keep a master set of all materials in case of accident or for further copying, and never circulate the masters. In putting the package together remember the user, and the individuals responsible for its care and distribution. If it is easy for them to use, they will be more inclined to do so. Remember that although your programme may have been designed for and produced in one medium, it is possible to distribute it in a variety of ways. For example, a slide-tape programme can be presented with a dissolve projection unit and recorded on videotape for convenient, always perfectly synchronised presentations.

Finally, allow plenty of time for preparing a programme: it may take longer than you expect. Nevertheless, it may relieve you of much repetitious lecturing and allow you time to have more useful and rewarding contact with your students.

And as a postscript: review your programme periodically and make sure it is up to date and able to achieve the objectives of current users.

Further reading

Baker, S. *Practical stylist (3rd Edn)*. New York: T Y Crowell, 1973.

Conway, J K, and Gilder, R S. *Medical and Biological Illustration* 1976; **26**: 167.

Engel, C E. *Medical and Biological Illustration* 1971; **21**: 14.

Evans, E M, and Eldridge, W S. *J Audiovisual Media Med* 1978; **1**: 140.

Gunning, R. *Techniques of clear writing*. New York: McGraw-Hill, 1968.

Harden, R McG, Wayne, E J, and Donald, G. *Medical and Biological Illustration*, 1968; **18**: 29.

Johnson, R B, and Johnson, S R. *Assuring learning with self-instructional packages, or up the up staircase*. Chapel Hill, Self Instructional Packages Inc, 1971.

Keckan, M. Producing an in-house video program. In: van Son, L G, ed. *Video in health*. White Plains, New York: Knowledge Industry Publications, 1982.

McArthur, J R. Conventional and high-technology teaching methods for educating health professionals in developing nations. *J Audiovisual Media Med* 1983; **6**: 43–4.

Prepare a patient education leaflet

J A MUIR GRAY

Few patients remember all that the doctor has said to them during a consultation. Patients usually remember those parts of the consultation that were most important to them but this does not necessarily include the points in the consultation that the doctor believed to be most important. Many patients are therefore unable to recollect all the advice they were given about treatment and self care.

The verbal aspect of the consultation has its limitations as a medium for transmitting information but the effectiveness of communication can be improved by complementing the spoken word with the written—by giving the patient a summary of what the doctor regards as the most important facts. Ideally, each patient would be given a written summary of the key points that had been covered in the consultation but this is rarely possible and a leaflet which summarises the main points that are of relevance to all patients with a particular problem offers a reasonable compromise to the doctor who would like to give his patients some written material but who is unable to write a different set of notes for each and every patient.

Why do it?

Before wondering how to do it, ask yourself—"Why do it?" Why prepare a leaflet yourself when there are numerous leaflets available?[1] Your local health education unit should be able to provide information on the leaflets that are available and perhaps provide samples or batches of them, but leaflets and booklets for patients and the public are now produced from so many sources that it is difficult for a health education unit to keep up to date. Other useful sources of information on patient education are the relevant mutual aid groups, for example the Alzheimer's Disease Society or the Parkinson's Disease Society or the community health council. The medical library in the postgraduate centre may be another very good source of information because many medical librarians are developing an interest in patient information and education.

Published leaflets are, in general, well produced and cheap; many are free. Some of them have been evaluated and most of those produced by drug companies are not used by them to push their own products offensively. There are, however, disadvantages about the use of published material, the principal one being that they have not been produced by the patient's own doctor, for, in spite of the adverse criticism of the medical profession which has become more vehement in recent years, the majority of patients still trust their own doctor's advice on health more than they trust advice from any other source. A stencilled sheet of advice produced by a patient's own doctor will usually be more effective than the glossiest leaflet produced by a third party because a leaflet, properly used, is not simply a vehicle for information; it can also symbolise the contract between doctor and patient, and thus be an extension and continuation of the consultation.

Writing a leaflet

Having decided to write a leaflet you have to decide on: content, length, language, style, and design.

Content

This may seem self evident but it is important to think of the objectives that are desired and to include relevant material for all the objectives. If, for example, the objectives are not only to inform but also to encourage a change in behaviour, specific information must be given on the appropriate behavioural change. Therefore ask yourself:

(1) What are the objectives of the leaflet?

(2) What needs to be put in to attain each of these objectives?

The content should include detailed specific advice and not simply vague exhortations. For example, instead of simply exhorting someone to "take more exercise," advice should be given on the frequency, duration, and intensity of exercise that will be beneficial.

Length

Brevity may be the soul of wit but it can also be the source of

174

confusion. Do not make the leaflet so brief that it is superficial or so general that it is ineffective. So much emphasis is put on the need to keep verbal messages short and simple that it is sometimes assumed that all forms of communication should be equally brief. But the patient will have time to read his leaflet at his leisure, and to return to it once, or many times, if he wishes, so it is possible to give more detail on particularly important points in a leaflet than when speaking to someone. This does not mean that a short book is justified, but one or two thousand words may be appropriate.

Language

The length chosen is inevitably a compromise, for most doctors have patients whose customary reading material ranges from the brevity of a racing card—the epitome of brief prose—to the prolixity of official documents. Similarly, the reading level of patients ranges from the ability to master only the shortest of words and the simplest of grammar—for example, the English found in tabloids—to the ability to cope with long words and sophisticated sentence structures—for example, the grammar of legal documents or government circulars. In the ideal world a range of different leaflets would be produced; in practice one leaflet must usually suffice. The compromise has to be written for the person who can cope with simple language but that compromise will be welcomed by most sophisticated patients, although a few will feel patronised.

Commonly used words are usually short and should be chosen in preference to longer words wherever possible. This is usually better English in any case; better to "use" a word than "employ" one. Sentences should also be short with as few subordinate clauses as possible. Take the *Daily Express* or *The Sun* for a few weeks if you are not a regular reader of a tabloid to read well written English of this sort.

Fowler's *Dictionary of Modern English Usage*[2] gives amusing and clear advice on the dangers of, and means of avoiding, "abstractitis" and the "love of the long word."

Style

Case histories, suitably disguised of course, increase the reader's interest and the question and answer format is also an effective style, particularly if the questions are those which patients commonly ask. The humorous approach is best avoided as humour often falls flat when translated to the written word.

Design

The design of a leaflet is important and the following possibilities should be considered:

- Diagrams
- Columns to reduce the length of lines
- Different type faces.

Patients who are printers, publishers, commercial artists, or designers will be able to offer good advice.

Remember to leave sufficient blank space on the leaflet for writing additional, personal, advice when giving the leaflet to the patient.

Theory into practice

The theory is comparatively simple: the practice of leaflet writing more difficult. But the doctor who is considering writing a leaflet should bear in mind two points—firstly, that his patients will greatly appreciate, and benefit from, such an initiative and, secondly, when starting to write to remember Robert Graves' famous dictum that a writer's best friend is his wastepaper basket. Do not attempt to achieve the perfect formula at the first attempt. Draft and redraft the text, viewing each draft as a step towards a useful working document.

Evaluation

Evaluation always improves effectiveness. Even very simple evaluation of a draft of the leaflet, for example by asking a small number of patients and other members of the primary care team for their comments, will improve the final version. The health visitor's training makes her a particularly useful critic or colleague if the topic is one that is of interest to her, and the health education unit is another very useful source of criticism and advice.

More formal evaluation is, of course, more effective and the district health authority's research fund or a relevant drug company are sources of finance for evaluation. The health education unit would be a good source of advice for drafting such a research application and one of the health education officers may be interested in participating in such a project.

The use of the leaflet

Leaflets which are left for patients to take have some effect but the leaflet is more valuable if used by a member of the primary care team in the course of his or her consultation with a patient. The leaflet should not simply be handed to the patient as he rises to leave but used during the consultation and at this stage it helps to personalise the leaflet, for example to write the patient's name on it, or underline parts of particular relevance to that patient or to write additional points in the spaces left for this purpose at the design stage. If the opportunity is also provided for the patient to record information on the leaflet the effectiveness will be further improved.

It is not easy to write an effective leaflet, but the effort is well worth making because a leaflet, properly prepared and used, can be a useful extension of the consultation.

[1] Sloan, P J M. Survey of patient information booklets. *Br Med J*, 1984; **288**: 915–19.
[2] Fowler, H. W. *A dictionary of modern English usage*. Oxford: OUP, 1926.

Produce a leaflet

PETER DORMER, JANE SMITH

In the beginning there is always the word: the difficulty is to persuade people to read it. Presentation and dissemination are vital. This chapter is aimed at the doctor who wants to produce a leaflet for his patients, a newsletter, or, if the need and the money exist, a more elaborate booklet. We have considered three broad options: the cheap, do-it-yourself approach using an IBM (or similar quality) typewriter or wordprocessor printer and the university or hospital offset litho machine; using the local "instant print" shop; and finding a designer and using a regular typesetter/printer.

But first ask what purpose the leaflet or newsletter is to serve, think hard about the target audience, and then decide on the format. (If you engage a designer he or she will ask you these questions.) Before considering questions of design and printing it is essential to be clear about the copy—the words. What is it to say? Indeed, what language should it be in? In many areas leaflets aimed at patients may need to be printed in Urdu or Gujarati as well as English (and that means finding a native speaker to translate and a typesetter who holds the relevant typefaces).

Deciding what has to be said is important because then you know the length of the copy in advance of the design and can judge, preferably in collaboration with a designer, what size the leaflet or newsletter should be, what typeface should be used, how it should be laid out, and whether illustrations should be included. Knowing these aspects in advance will result in a better presentation and means that a realistic budget can be established.

Conversely, if you know you can afford (or want) to produce only, say, a four page A5 leaflet then that will determine how much you can say—a good discipline but harder work.

Doing it yourself

In the do-it-yourself approach you are acting as your own typesetter and compositor. The method is cheap but may be time consuming. It requires a good quality electric typewriter or wordprocessor printer and access to an offset litho machine. Many organisations—especially those producing a lot of paperwork—have in house printing departments with platemaking facilities and small offset litho machines, usually run by a specialist operator who may also provide advice. For design, we assume that at this level you are relying on your own or a colleague's flair.

At its simplest you can merely type, neatly and without mistakes, the copy on to a page of A4 typing paper and reproduce that. For a large number of copies offset litho is cheaper than photocopying and better looking than duplicated sheets produced from a stencil. The plate making stage of lithography usually offers the possibility of reduction, so four typewritten sheets of A4 paper could, for example, be reduced and compiled into a four page A5 leaflet.

If you want something more elaborate, perhaps including diagrams, you can type sections of the text, cut them out, and paste them down on a clean sheet of paper together with any illustrations and any separate titles and headings. The advantage of using an IBM golfball typewriter is that the typefaces are interchangeable. Some IBM and other electric typewriters and wordprocessor printers can justify text as well. (Justified text has straight margins on both sides; unjustified has a ragged edge on the right.) Just because various typefaces are available you don't have to use all of them at once. Keep things simple, or the result will be a mess. The same applies to headings and titles.

If you want more distinctive headings than those offered by typewriter faces you can use Letraset or a similar rub down transfer lettering. These come in a wide range of typefaces and sizes and you should consult the catalogue before choosing. Do not automatically go for capitals: capital letters often make boring headings that are harder to read than a mixture of upper and lower case letters. Good office or graphic art shops sell Letraset and will have the catalogues. Using these lettering systems has its drawbacks, however. Transfer lettering is expensive and, for the novice, time consuming to apply. The pitfalls are getting the spacing right between the letters and keeping the line of lettering straight. A drawing board with a fixed horizontal rule is essential, as indeed it is for any work that involves pasting down separate items straight on a sheet of paper and drawing straight lines. Resist the temptation to go wild with the Letraset: keep it unpretentious.

Line drawings—cartoons or diagrams drawn in black ink on

white paper with no shading—are as easy to reproduce as the typewritten letters and may add greatly to the usefulness and look of a leaflet or newsletter. But drawings with shading, or photographs, present additional problems and should probably be avoided at the do it yourself level.

Look at (and borrow from) other leaflets or publications that serve a similar purpose to yours. Look at the layout and typeface of the display lettering (the titles and headings), the distribution of paragraphs, and the tabulations of facts and figures. Do not be afraid of leaving open space: good designs often have a lot of "air" in them.

Emphasise a single fact or concept by putting the key sentence in a larger type, by isolating it, or by juxtaposing it with an illustration. Letraset and others produce sheets of transfer patterns, lines, and decorations. Used sparingly they can add interest to a page of text. But, again, do not overdo the tricks.

"Instant printing"

All this can, of course, be done without an in house offset litho machine. You can take your artwork—for that is what you have produced—instead to the high street instant print shop (see Yellow Pages) and get them to print it for you—at a few pounds per page per thousand copies. Alternatively, you can get the print shop to produce the entire leaflet for you, because many offer design and typesetting as well as printing. They will show you samples, help you select a typeface, find out whether you want illustrations or more than one colour, and produce a rough design for your approval. They will then set it, lay it out, and print it.

By using a typesetting and paste up service you are freed straight away from the "typewriter" look and from the time consuming business of producing artwork. For straightforward one or two colour work folded and bound simply and for ephemera such as handbills, tickets, and letterheadings the print shop will usually provide reasonable quality at a reasonable cost. All you need to do is know what you want, how much you can afford, and supply clean copy and any relevant illustrations.

Clean copy is neatly typed text with very few corrections and clearly marked instructions on items like headings. Dirty copy puts the price up. If you are having anything set by any sort of typesetter you will be shown proofs, which need reading carefully and correcting as necessary (proof correction marks are printed in *Whitaker's Almanack*). Errors made by the typesetter will be corrected at no charge to the author, but if you start rewriting your text at proof stage costs will escalate.

Using a designer and printer

If you have money and want to produce something that has a lot of illustrations, for example, or is specially bound, then commission a designer. He or she will produce a design that fits your requirements. The designer can specify everything affecting the visual presentation of your material—from the form of your publication to the type of paper and the cover and type of binding: he or she will produce roughs for your approval and then go on to produce final layouts with specifications of typeface and size. He can also select the typesetter/printer and be responsible for the quality of production (this is particularly important if you are including colour work). If you want the designer to prepare artwork and commission photography and illustrations this will cost more. Before commissioning a designer be clear about what you are asking him or her to do and get estimates of the costs.

If you want to produce anything other than the simplest of leaflets then find a designer. If you are starting a newsletter you can ask the designer to design the first issue and lay down a style for subsequent issues. You will then know what typeface and size to mark up for the printer and can ask the printer to paste up subsequent issues according to the page layout set by the designer. This does mean that the editor will have to know how to calculate the space that his copy will fill and know how to size illustrations and so forth (see bibliography).

There are several ways of finding a designer. If you see a brochure or magazine you like inquire about its designer from the publisher or printer. But designers specialise too, and the designer of a slick company report may not be the best person to design the local medical society's newsletter. You may also contact the local art college (usually part of a polytechnic) and ask for the names of good new graduates in graphic or typographic design, or offer your leaflet to the graphics department as a student project (they will probably be keen if the leaflet is aimed at patients, and you may get your design for free). For prestige work contact the Design Council, the Society of Industrial Artists and Designers, or the Society of Typographic Designers (addresses below). From these lists of names you can select two or three and ask to see their work.

Many typesetting and printing companies have in house designers and offer designing as well as setting and printing. Many are capable but cannot do what an independent designer may so—shop around to find the most suitable typesetter and printer. Nevertheless, you can select two or three printers (if you do not know any look in the Yellow Pages), ask them for quotations, and ask to see examples of their designs. Finding a printer who will also do the design is often the easiest solution, especially if your intended publication is simple and you have a small budget.

We have avoided discussing the use of full colour illustrations because these are expensive to print, and design advice is essential to get the best effect from colour.

In essence if you know what you want to say there should be no difficulty in getting your words well presented. A little research and planning and your words will carry wherever you want them to go.

Note

The law requires that anything published in the United Kingdom—that is, anything produced other than for internal circulation—must carry the name and address of the printer and/or publisher—usually on the last page. A professional printer will have his own form of words for this imprint and should include it automatically. If you are preparing your own artwork for the office offset litho, however, you must remember to include this information.

Design Coucil, 28 Haymarket, London SW1.
Society of Industrial Artists and Designers, 12 Carlton House Terrace, London SW1.
Society of Typographic Designers, Highbury Crescent, London N5.

McLean, R. *The Thames and Hudson manual of typography*. London: Thames and Hudson, 1980.
Murray, R. *How to brief designers and buy print*. London: Business Books, 1983.
Treweek, C, Zeithyn, J, and with the Islington Bus Company. *The alternative printing handbook*. Harmondsworth, Middlesex: Penguin, 1983.

182

Use a library

MORAG C TIMBURY, SHEILA E CANNELL,
MARGARET M COUTTS

All doctors must be familiar with libraries from their student days although not all will continue to use a library regularly throughout their career. However, the emphasis nowadays on the need for continuing education together with the pressure to publish make it likely that the use of medical libraries will increase. We are exceptionally lucky in Britain in that we have numerous large libraries situated in universities, colleges, and research institutions. Even doctors who do not live near a major centre can obtain medical literature via the excellent postal service of the BMA library in Tavistock Square, London.

Most of us who use libraries a lot probably do not encounter any particular problems, but even regular visits may well not reveal the wealth of material and resources available. The best advice an article like this can give is to contact the library staff. This can save a great deal of time quite apart from the benefit of professional help in getting to know the full potential of the library facilities. Library staff enjoy guiding readers to the literature sought as well as the occasional challenge of finding some esoteric piece of information.

Depending on the circumstances, most of us will use different categories of information sources at some time, or indeed many times in our careers. These sources can be broadly defined as:

(1) Current periodicals
(2) Review articles and textbooks
(3) Reference books.

Current periodicals

Large libraries have hundreds of current journals and those not stocked can be obtained by interlibrary loan from the British Library Lending Division at Boston Spa. In days gone by a literature search consisted of looking up the references quoted in a

183

key article and then, in widening circles, the secondary references in the articles quoted and so on. This would be complemented by a manual search of *Index Medicus*—still an invaluable reference source. Modern computer technology has revolutionised this. Now a list of relevant articles (with authors, titles, and sources) can be quickly obtained by a Medline search. Medline is MEDLARS online (Medical Literature Analysis and Retrieval System). Based on the subject headings (MeSH) in *Index Medicus*, the search is qualified by subheadings such as "aetiology" and "therapy" to reduce the printout to manageable proportions. The list of periodicals covered goes back to 1966 although most often the search is limited to the preceding four years. Although in Britain we have not, for the most part, had to pay for our information, some libraries charge for Medline searches. The average cost is between £5·00 and £20·00 but this pays for itself in the saving in staff time and frustration. Medline facilities are widely available and most large hospital libraries now have them. There are also various specialised databases such as Cancerline, Psycinfo, and the delightfully named Popline, which has nothing to do with the Rolling Stones but covers the literature on population and family planning.

Another source of references is *Science Citation Index* although this one has some slightly sinister undertones. *Science Citation Index* has a subject index (permuterm) together with the citation index proper which lists the authors and their articles which have been quoted in the literature of the current year. The authors and articles in which the original author is cited are also listed. Its particular use is as a quick guide to relevant articles when the name of a key worker is known. However, it can also be a rough and ready yardstick of a worker's contribution to research in the sense that it lists authors and the frequency with which their articles are still being quoted in the literature. *Index to Scientific and Technical Proceedings* lists authors, titles and addresses of papers presented at meetings. Proceedings of scientific meetings are, of course, usually unrefereed and sometimes unedited but often contain the earliest report of an interesting development or breakthrough.

Abstract journals are a quick if rather indigestible way of keeping up to date with the literature. Numerous abstract journals are available but they tend to suffer from being slow and appear, for obvious reasons, much later than the original articles. Readers may not realise that abstracts can be obtained for something like 40% of the references on Medline. One popular version of the abstract is the Minerva column in the *British Medical Journal*. Although obviously not structured or systematic, it is an enjoyable read and draws attention to points of interest which have struck contributors (Minerva is, alas, neither completely female nor singular) from a wide field of medical publications.

Review articles and textbooks

A good monograph or review article is often the most efficient way of getting a balanced and detailed overview of a subject. Large numbers are published each year—some under titles like "Recent Advances" or "Annual Reviews." Like articles in periodicals, review articles are also listed in *Index Medicus*.

Libraries, of course, have large stocks of textbooks although the latest edition of the one wanted always seems to be out on loan. Readers often forget that books can be reserved and recalled—a service that librarians feel is underused.

Reference books

One of the most enjoyable ways to spend a quiet afternoon at work is a browse in the reference section of the local medical library. Medical readers not familiar with this section will be astonished at the breadth and depth of information available. Some of the bibliographies make enjoyable reading. One of our favourites is *Medical Eponyms: Who was Coudé* by J Lowrie, which gives short and entertaining biographies of the people whose names are immortalised in this way.Coudé is of course a trap: "he" is the French word for elbow. Another favourite is *The Harvest of a Quiet Eye* by A L Mackay: the title is a quotation from Wordsworth and obscures the fact that it is a delightful collection of medical quotations. *The Hospitals and Health Services Year Book* continues to be an astonishingly comprehensive source of information about the NHS, and hard pressed research workers looking for funds will find *The Directory of Grant-making Trusts* a helpful signpost.

New technology

Libraries have not been immune from new technology. Many libraries now have automated issue systems—but a terminal can be much less generous than the librarian behind the desk with overdue books. In some libraries the catalogue of books and periodicals will now be on computer. Don't be scared of these: the reader is not able to damage the information stored in the computers and they are much easier to use than traditional catalogues.

With new technology, the future of libraries may be very

different from what we know and love today. The reader may not even need to come to an actual library building, but may be able to read periodical articles, books, and reference books at his own desk, with the computer terminal or microcomputer which he also uses for word processing or laboratory work. He will read from the screen and only print out what he wants to keep as printed copy.

Already several significant periodicals and books are available in electronic format, including the *Lancet* and the *British Medical Journal*. By computer, a searcher keys in any word—for example, viruses—and the system will find and print all recent articles which contain the word anywhere in the text. In medicine, no major journal is yet published only in electronic format, but that may come soon as the economics of publishing sway in favour of electronic media. Current research projects are investigating the future pattern of periodical publishing: the medical community must monitor publishers closely to ensure the continuation of the quality refereed journals essential for their work.

Libraries will consequently have to change to encompass this new method of publishing: but despite the changes, the librarian, perhaps lurking under a different title of "information officer," will still be there to help the doctor find the information he wants, whether in a book or on a computer.

How not to use a library

Unfortunately, no article of this sort can ignore the negative side of library use. Librarians are well aware that otherwise honest and upright citizens occasionally show no apparent qualms of conscience about "removing" books. In large libraries the supervision is now such that entry occasionally seems harder than breaking into Fort Knox and one of us has had difficulty in retaining an admittedly large handbag. Perhaps not surprisingly these Gestapo-like measures have not totally succeeded in stopping thefts. The even more heinous crime of tearing out a favourite or key article should now have ceased with the increasing availability of photocopies but apparently still goes on albeit on a reduced scale. A word of caution is necessary about photocopying because libraries and other public bodies are taking a much tougher line on copyright law. This restricts copying, for example, to only one article per issue of a periodical for private study or research. New staff members and students of this university must now sign a declaration that they will not contravene the copyright law. Despite obvious difficulties in detection, it seems certain that prosecutions for copyright infringement will increase.

Conclusion

This article has been written by two professional librarians and an enthusiastic amateur. Of necessity we have omitted to mention many other useful library services and facilities—notably those of small departmental libraries most of which have suffered badly in the university cuts. Communication is becoming ever more sophisticated and important in all walks of life and certainly so in medicine. Doctors can only gain from learning to make the best use of the excellent medical libraries we are fortunate to have here in Britain.

Further reading

Morton L T, Godbolt S, eds. *Information services in the medical sciences*, 3rd ed. London: Butterworth, 1984.

Be a dictator

HEATHER WINDLE

Despite the proliferation of word processors and computers capable of handling routine letters, doctors still find it necessary to dictate one-off letters, papers, reports and so on. Word processors, incidentally, have dangers: a sentence may carelessly be changed without the rest of the text being checked for inconsistencies, and mistakes are often repeated ad infinitum. It is as well to remember that a computer lacks imagination and its brain is limited by the quality of the data fed in by man. Even so, they are now becoming addictive and many a doctor has become hooked on a computer. Although, for example, Ritchie[1] thinks that general practitioners are more likely to want a computer in the reception area than in the consulting room I suspect that a small desktop microcomputer with a visual display unit may prove irresistible to many and will have an unexpected side effect: the doctor concerned will have to learn to type if he is to dictate to his computer.

The operator's newly acquired skill will not, however, mean that he will type his own letters; he will undoubtedly need someone else to cope with his correspondence and papers, but I hope will use his computer for referral and recall letters, letters to insurance companies and employers so that he (or she) can make the best use of his secretary or shorthand or audio typist. One or two doctors have mentioned to me how inadequate they feel when confronted by an efficient looking girl (or, less usually, a man) with a notebook and a pencil poised expectantly waiting for him or her to begin speaking. What can they do to overcome their nervousness, they ask. No doubt the answer is to have confidence in their knowledge about the matter to be dictated but they seem to be more concerned about technique. I may be able to help because during a particularly horrendous period in my life when my children were at school I worked as a temporary secretary for some 200–300 different men (99% *were* men, but with equal oportunities for all no doubt the percentage has gone down, particularly in the medical world). During that time I encountered practically every good and bad type of personality in man, and every possible vagary in typewriter, taperecorder, and other machines, for which I had little natural aptitude. My sympathies, therefore, are primarily with the person on the receiving end of dictation but I admit to a little experience on the other side of the fence, which was almost as difficult because I was young at the time and my secretary was old.

You may dictate direct or into a dictating machine or taperecorder, and both have advantages and disadvantages. If you are doing it by remote control—for example, a consultant who goes to a hospital once a week, dictates into a machine, and signs the finished letters a week later—then presumably you will continue on this antisocial course. If you dictate direct or have any other communication with the secretary or shorthand or audio typist, however, please call her (even nowadays it is usually a woman) by her name—let's say it is Jane—and treat her as if she is as clever, or almost as clever, as you. She won't be a doctor but, unknown to you, may have a first in English or an IQ of 140; she will be more willing to stop you making mistakes if you take advantage of at least some of her talents. You may both find a mixture of shorthand and dictating machine the best way to manage work that may be dictated during office hours or outside them.

Jane should be able to write some letters herself if you give her a rough outline of what you want to say. Let her do as much as she is capable of, because that will retain her interest better than routine dictation. If you treat her well she will do much for you—as well as correcting your grammar, she may remind you about unanswered or forgotten letters, or point out mistakes you're making in other ways. A great deal, however, will have to be done by dictation.

Shorthand

Shorthand has great advantages. You or Jane can correct letters easily as you go along or afterwards if they are longwinded or rubbish, and Jane can tell you when you've repeated yourself. Make sure she has a suitable chair and a typewriter that works properly. She may be nervous, so collect your thoughts and the day's work together (if possible, dictate in one or two batches, but not for too long at a stretch, and then leave her in peace), and, if you are a muddler, make a few notes to guide you (and give the notes to Jane when you've finished). You should be able to judge the best speed to dictate by whether Jane looks frantic or bored—in time, her speed will increase to match yours, but take it easy to start with. If you can restrain yourself, punctuate only when essential because punctuation distracts, and you shouldn't have to make her read the whole thing back.

When answering letters give Jane the originals and do not dictate the address. Spell out difficult words—drugs and diseases, for example—and don't say "Dear Bimbo" without indicating who he is. Correcting typed letters in ink is maddening; Jane may prefer to change mistakes neatly herself (particularly if they are her own). You should take advantage of your contact with her. If you want her to stay on ask her sometimes for her opinion. She will be flattered and you may be surprised to find that she has useful ideas about speeches and articles.

Recording machines

Tape recorders come in many different makes, and it is easy to forget how to use one, even after a short time. Jane should have a foot pedal and earphones, and she should not be surrounded by tripwires. One snag about recording is that people tend to like the sound of their own voices, letters become prolix, and addressees merely scan them and perhaps miss the point. So keep them short, and do give Jane an idea of the length. Another snag is second thoughts; nothing is more irritating than to hear half way through: "Sorry, scrub the first paragraph." You can easily erase the tape and start again. Remember, Jane will have to type the letters exactly as she hears them so don't be surprised if they are returned to you looking like the writings of an illiterate schoolboy—she has little chance of correcting them when they are on tape and she certainly does not want to hear it more than once—even deathless prose becomes boring if repeated too often. Another, and more serious, snag is the time it takes for an overworked audiotypist to tackle a tape. Once you've dictated something it's easy to forget that it hasn't come back for signature. This hardly ever happens with shorthand.

Many girls prefer to be separated from their bosses by machines, but there is still room for the personal touch. If you mention Jane's name on the tape sometimes, if only to say "Good morning, Jane," or "Jane, please remind me about that," it makes all the difference to a good working partnership, but fatuous remarks about the test match or the weather go down less well.

Points to remember

Dictating in the street, car, nursery, plane, or train makes transcribing difficult for Jane when she has to sort out your words from children's cries, traffic sounds, or Bach.

If you and Jane have different mother tongues or idioms (Americans can be as difficult as Greeks or Romans) dictate slowly and, if necessary, repeat words with a different emphasis—otherwise the words will still be double Dutch to her. If you can't spell, employ someone who can (have a list of words to try out on her), or you may become the object of ridicule. (My daughter and a publisher boss of hers sent out hundreds of letters about "soul distribution rights" before they were spotted.) And don't wander about away from the microphone or out of the room while you're dictating or chunks will be missing from your letters.

One word about speeches: write down an outline before dictating because you may lose the thread, and give the notes to Jane. Normally, you should be willing to answer her questions (better for her to ask than get it wrong), but with a speech she may be reluctant to interrupt you.

There are other ways of dictating, most of them torture. You may dictate to Jane over the telephone and not visualise her desk covered in papers, another telephone ringing, people interrupting her, and her shorthand book balanced on the typewriter while hanging on to the telephone with the other hand. If you must do that, buy one of the machines that holds the receiver and amplifies the voice—thus leaving both Jane's hands free. Taking down shorthand in a car is difficult too: the car lurches round a corner, Jane and her book slither across the seat, and you're still holding forth as before.

I have concentrated on how to be a dictator and omitted the more subtle secretarial side of Jane's job, but, whether she's a secretary or a typist, you should treat her with patience and consideration, talk with her sometimes rather than at her, remember her birthday, and don't treat her as if she's half witted. If you're nice to her she'll put up with you when you're irritable, forgetful, unreasonable, overbearing, or drunk, but, remember, it's not *fun* taking down your dictation—it's a job—so try to make the job as interesting for her as you can. If you trust her, and you should not employ her if you don't, you may even be able to grant her access to your computer with a codeword of her own; then she will be able to handle some of the data more accurately than you do and also be spared some of the drudgery of her own work.

---

[1] Ritchie, Lewis D. *Computers in primary care.* London: William Heinemann Medical Books, 1984.

Choose a microcomputer

A J ASBURY

Start by ignoring the persuasive salesmen and colourful magazine advertisements and decide in broad terms what you want the computer to do for you. For example do you just want to learn about computers or do you want it to help you write your MD thesis, manage the practice accounts, or do the calculations for your research project. Bear in mind the fact that most people underspecify what they want, and many make false assumptions. For example, have you assumed that a suitable printed record will necessarily be available with the computer that you buy? The more accurately you specify your needs, the more likely you are to buy the right computer.

The library is now the next stop, where you should look out books and journals on basic computing applied to microcomputers. Your reading will help you further define your requirements and introduce you to computing concepts and terminology.

Now get some unbiased help to translate your requirements into a real computer description. It is particularly important with specialised applications to talk to somebody who really understands your application. If, for example, you are a general practitioner buying a computer for general practice why not consult the RCGP computer experts, and, most important, visit a GP who is actually using a computer in general practice. You might well decide that a computer is more trouble than it is worth. In addition a local university computing department will usually provide unbiased advice and welcomes discussions with potential computer users.

Memory

Here the link between the application and the computer becomes important. If you are mainly interested in learning programming youself, or perhaps teaching the children, then it is

192

unlikely that you will need more than 32 kilobytes of random access memory (RAM). Most people, however, buy a computer and do a small amount of programming themselves, and also use ready made programs (packages). If you intend to use the computer to run packages—for example data storage, statistics, administration, games, accounting, or word processing, then you must make sure that not only do you buy the right computer for the package, but that the right computer has enough memory for the package.

One pitfall regarding memory size is that some manufacturers state the amount of memory, implying that it is all available for the program. In reality only a fraction may be available in certain modes, as the computer uses some to support the graphics displays.

Graphics and computer display

Graphics facilities, the ability of the computer to specify the colour and intensity of a small part (pixel) of the display screen, have revolutionsed computer use and spawned the highly profitable video games industry. Graphics are now increasingly being used in teaching—for example, to draw graphs and animate simulations. On the debit side graphics facilities may reduce the memory available to the user to write his programs.

If graphics facilities are required, then one must have a suitable display. A standard domestic colour television may be totally inadequate for fine details, and a separate colour monitor would be necessary. A good high resolution colour monitor can cost as much as the computer itself.

One trend in computing is to simplify the "human-computer interface," by providing a pictorial representation of the operating system. If you wish, for example, to open a file, then you manoeuvre the cursor over the screen image of the open file (called an ikon), and the computer does the rest. There are several methods of moving the cursor, the obvious being to press the relevant keys. A newer technique is to employ a joystick, or a "mouse," both of which allow one handed control of the cursor. One manufacturer has produced a computer with a touch sensitive screen, and you merely need to touch the relevant ikon with your finger.

The keyboard

If you are planning to use the computer for much more than games then you need a full size keyboard; this is particularly

193

important if you intend to do word processing, as calculator style keyboards make text entry very slow.

Storing information

In most micros when the power is disconnected, the text, programs, results, etc, in the random access memory (RAM) are lost. To retain the memory contents you must store them in another way, and the commonest method is to store it on a ferromagnetic medium. Magnetic tape on cassettes is an obvious choice, being cheap and readily available. The problem with tape is that information retrieval can be slow and sometimes unreliable. On the other hand, many companies distribute programs on cassette tape.

Flexible (floppy) disc storage is a faster, more reliable, but more expensive method of information storage. Discs vary in diameter from 3 to 8 inches and can hold up to two million characters. The major trap for the buyer is that each disc unit manufacturer has a different system for storing the information on the disc, and one should not assume that a discful of information written on to a disc by one computer will necessarily be readable by another.

Hard disc storage allows storage of even more information than floppy discs—often up to ten million characters—with very fast access times. Unfortunately hard disc units are expensive and not readily portable. Some recent computers feature a built-in hard disc unit.

Printers

There are two main forms of printer. The daisywheel printer produces text similar in quality and form to that of a good typewriter. Daisywheel printers are usually slow, taking perhaps a minute to print a page of text. Dot matrix printers are noisier, faster, and frequently cheaper than daisywheel printers, but the print quality is poorer, each letter being formed from a series of dots. Matrix printers are, however, very flexible—for example, it is possible to change type font and colour on a document without stopping or making adjustments to the printer.

The main trap for the buyer lies in the consumables—that is, paper, dairywheels, and ribbons. These seemingly small items can become very expensive, particularly with word processing. Make sure that the printer takes the type of paper or forms that you want to use and that it will be able to feed into the printer automatically. Some elegant printers require special papers—for example, heat sensitive papers, which are very expensive, and the mechanism of the printer will not allow you to use any other. Check that the consumables are actually readily available and at a reasonable price.

Communications

Many manufacturers make computers with built-in facilities for communicating over telephone lines. This enables the user to access data collections, such as PRESTEL, programs, and notices held on larger computers remote from the user. A very useful facility is to be able to collect data locally and, after suitable editing, transmit it to a central computer which has better data handling facilities.

Final decisions

Having defined one's requirements, the field should have narrowed considerably. Now is the time to scan the relevant journals and look for reviews dealing with your shortlisted computers; if necessary take the reviews and discuss them with your long suffering expert. It is worth finding out where your favoured few stand in the market, and asking questions such as: Is the market price due to fall soon? Is it due to be superseded by another model? Are parts likely to be avilable? Is it reliable? Is the documentation good? Is there a local user group nearby? Some companies run a phone-in service for their users, and, though you obviously pay for such convenience, it can, like good documentation, save you time.

Now you know what you want, consult the journals and seek the most favourable "deal." You may be able to negotiate a reduced price by buying all your requirements through one dealer, but ensure that this does not compromise your guarantee. It is also worth checking your VAT status as the regulations are changing all the time. You may be exempt from VAT in your particular application.

Many manufacturers advertise the price of the "bare system" without cables, documentation, etc, so check precisely what you get for your money.

It is often convenient to buy your chosen computer via a magazine advertisement, but there can be disadvantages. Suppose that you send your money and the goods are not delivered in a reasonable time. The company may be holding on to your money "until stocks arrive," and this might take some time. It could be that your requirements were not very specific and that your second choice would be equally suitable and readily available down the road. If you are dealing at long distance you cannot easily apply pressure on the supplier. The same reasoning applies to getting your equipment serviced. Things always take longer if you have to send the apparatus away by post, compared with visiting your local dealer. If you do send your computer away for repair, don't forget to insure it.

Now reach for your chequebook.

Choose and use a calculator

T D V SWINSCOW

A potential customer looking at the glittering ranks of calculators in a shop window is apt to be amazed at the wonders of science. This is the shopkeeper's intention. The object of this article is to reduce the bewilderment that may supervene.

Choosing a calculator

The first question a doctor, like any other customer, should begin by asking himself is what purposes his calculator must serve. Is it to do the household accounts, for example, or his daughter's A level maths, metric conversions, arithmetical computations related to his practice, or correlation coefficients? Many individual calculators can perform all these functions and more, but so many specialised models are now available that if a restricted function is intended for it a calculator designed for that purpose is worth getting. In fact anyone who uses a calculator frequently will probably find that he needs more than one. The first may be a convenient little calculator for doing simple sums, the second a more elaborate or specialised machine. One may be "slim line" and carried in the pocket, another larger for the desk top. And, as often in life, it pays to buy the best. That generally means, with calculators, avoiding the cheapest. There are plenty on the market that are unreliable and short-lived owing to shoddy workmanship. Be prepared therefore to pay more than the minimum.

The potential user will find that there are two main systems by which calculators are operated, and he may wonder which to opt for. One is known as "algebraic logic," the other as "reverse Polish notation." Most calculators work on algebraic logic, and they are sometimes marketed with the claim, expressed or implied, that they are more "natural" to use and therefore easier. Algebraic logic

197

deals with calculations in the same order as we say them. In $2 + 3 = 5$, for example, keys are successively pressed for 2, $+$, 3, and $=$. In the reverse Polish notation there is no key for $=$. Instead there is a key marked Enter, and the above addition is done as follows: 2, Enter, 3, $+$. The answer then appears. This order of working is in fact akin to how we do a sum on paper, and it comes perfectly readily after a little practice. Each system has advantages. Some users might find difficulty in switching from one to the other and so, if they own several calculators, prefer to have all in the same mode, but in practice to go from one mode to the other is not a serious problem.

What is much more likely to cause trouble is to use calculators made by different manufacturers. Calculators that look alike but are of different makes are apt to produce divergent results from the same series of operations. For example, on two of my calculators I may carry out the following computation: $2 + 3 \times 4$. On the first calculator the answer is 20, that is, $(2 + 3) \times 4$; on the second it is 14, that is, $2 + (3 \times 4)$. These and some other differences that I have tested are consistent between other models of these two manufacturers. No doubt each manufacturer fits a certain type of computation into his range of models, and it commonly differs in some respects from what his rivals provide.

Even cheap instruments nowadays provide a memory, and this facility is well worth having whatever the calculator's purpose. It saves writing down intermediate stages of calculations. Some calculators have more than one memory, so that the results of several stages in a long calculation can be stored. Another facility of this kind is the provision of parentheses within which a subsidiary calculation can be carried out, the result of which is then combined with the result of a previous calculation. This is a useful addition but not perhaps so essential as a memory. A "continuous memory" that stores its contents even after the instrument is switched off, so that they remain to be used in further calculations later on, is a further refinement sometimes offered.

Until recently few calculators were particularly suitable for the kind of statistical operations that doctors are likely to carry out— for example, standard deviation, chi-square test, product moment correlation, and regression equations. But now several can be found at two levels of complexity. The first offers in addition to the basic functions listed above a key for x^2 and $\sqrt{x}$. With a calculator so equipped the ordinary statistical computations are quickly carried out. The second type provides keys that save time on some of these computations, so that pressing one key will give the standard deviation, for example. It is important if buying one of these to check the formula used.

198

They work on the identity

$$\Sigma(\bar{x} - x)^2 = \Sigma x^2 - \frac{(\Sigma x)^2}{n}.$$

To calculate the variance (= square of standard deviation) it is necessary to divide this expression by $n - 1$. Calculators that divide by n should be rejected.

Having got so far, the potential customer will find that many calculators are now offered with a facility for inserting a set of instructions, or "program" (so spelt), that the machine will operate automatically. These are well worth investigating to see how any special needs the user may have in mind can be met. For example, many types of laboratory calculations as well as those required in statistical testing could be simplified by means of standard programs. Here it is worth emphasising that calculators are much better bought from shops that specialise in them rather than from stationers, chemists, photographers, and so on. Some specialist shops have well informed and expert staff who can give much more detailed advice than can be put into an article of this kind.

Just as cars, microscopes, and forceps have physical properties that please or vex their owners, so do calculators. Though they all look much alike, they handle very differently—for instance, in some the keys give a small click when depressed, while in others they provide little or no sensation to the finger tip. My own preference is for a distinct sensation of finality to the pressure put on the key. Incidentally, when trying out the feel of the keys it is worth pressing firmly on those round the periphery to make sure that the instrument is stable, for some tend to tip up.

Nearly all calculators nowadays have a liquid crystal display activated by a small battery lasting a year or more. The numbers are even less visible than on the older illuminated display. In sunlight and in twilight they become elusive and in darkness, of course, disappear.

Using a calculator

The manufacturers of calculators provide their customers with instruction books, but many have not taken the trouble to ensure that their authors are literate as well as numerate. Here, for example, is what the handbook of one calculator tells us about what it calls its "auto-constant mode": "The first factor of multiply and the second factor of addition, subtraction, and division are stored by the calculator logic after execution is complete." The handbooks are full of this kind of stuff (often in several languages), and I believe that a reader who fails to understand it at his first attempt need not blame his education. But unfortunately he must persevere, calculator in hand, because it is all he will get. There are no general rules for the use of calculators, for different models vary in all sorts of tricky computational details, some of which are discovered only after considerable experience. For example, an instrument I use has a parentheses facility, but some operations such as $\sqrt{x}$ cannot be carried out within the parentheses—a limitation, incidentally, not mentioned in the handbook.

In fact, after working through the handbook's instructions and practising them on his calculator the novice would be well advised to try out all sorts of further calculations. He will find that the handbook may fail to tell him of some that are possible as well as of others that are impossible on his particular instrument. The following type of calculation, for instance, is commonly needed: A series of numbers add up to a total. What percentage of the total is each number? $51 + 42 + 37 = 130$; percentages $39 \cdot 2 + 32 \cdot 3 + 28 \cdot 5 = 100$. By using the same constant, for example, $\dfrac{100}{130} \times$, it is easy to cut down the amount of computation needed. But each of the two calculators I use requires a different series of operations to do this, and neither's handbook gives any guidance on them.

Again, it is sometimes necessary to divide the displayed number into another number, that is, to use the display as a divisor. On some of the smaller calculators this is impossible. On others the following operation (not necessarily described in the instruction manual) will succeed: x (on the display) $\div = \times$ n. This achieves $\dfrac{n}{x}$ by computing $\dfrac{1}{x} \times n$.

Many calculators limit the display to eight digits, though some have facilities (varying from one model to another) of handling numbers with more digits. But the user needs to beware of losing the significant digits beyond the bounds of his instrument. In statistical calculations, where squares can quickly produce surprisingly large or small numbers, it is important to ensure that the significant digits are within bounds. And while very large and small numbers can obviously cause trouble, quite ordinary numbers may do so too if the differences between them are relatively small.

The example of this given below is taken from *Statistics at square one*.[1] The standard deviation of the following numbers is computed on an eight-digit calculator: $64 \cdot 22, 64 \cdot 23, 64 \cdot 24, 64 \cdot 25, 64 \cdot 27$. Here $\Sigma x = 321 \cdot 21$, $n = 5$, $(\Sigma x)^2 = 103175 \cdot 86$, $(\Sigma x)^2/n = 20635 \cdot 172$, Σx^2

$= 20635 \cdot 172$, $\Sigma(\bar{x} - x)^2 = 0$, $SD = 0$. But since the numbers differ from each other they must have a standard deviation.

What is needed here is to get the size of each number nearer to the differences between them. If 64 is subtracted from each we get $0 \cdot 22$, $0 \cdot 23$, $0 \cdot 24$, $0 \cdot 25$, $0 \cdot 27$. These give $\Sigma x = 1 \cdot 21$, $n = 5$, $(\Sigma x)^2 = 1 \cdot 4641$, $(\Sigma x)^2/n = 0 \cdot 29282$, $\Sigma x^2 = 0 \cdot 2943$, $\Sigma(\bar{x} - x)^2 = 0 \cdot 00148$, $\Sigma(\bar{x} - x)^2/(n - 1) = 0 \cdot 00037$, $SD = 0 \cdot 0192353$, which can be rounded off to $0 \cdot 02$.

A general rule, therefore, is to watch the significant digits in any calculation. If they get far away from unity, whether very large or very small, a simple transformation to cut them down to manageable size should be considered.

As well as respecting the limits of a calculator it is worth remembering that the human brain is not inexhaustible. Boring and repetitive calculations are tiring and can lead to errors from carelessness or sheer fatigue. A telephone call from a patient or an unexpected visitor from Porlock can likewise cause the operator to press the wrong key or lose track of the calculation. To guard against this I often write down the intermediate results of a laborious calculation, even such a simple one as adding up long columns of figures. I jot down, for instance, the sum of each column separately or the cumulative sums: column 1, columns $1 + 2$, columns $1 + 2 + 3$, and so on. This procedure helps the operator to carry out the final and most important part of his calculations, and that is to check them.

Always check the calculations. Check them right through, and check them if possible in a different order from the first set of calculations.

[1] Swinscow, T D V. *Statistics at square one*, 8th ed. London: British Medical Association, 1983.

Present numerical results

T D V SWINSCOW

Two fairly distinct kinds of articles with numerical data appear in medical journals. The aim of the first is primarily educational. The author is not putting forward any original, novel, or unusual material. He is trying to present his ideas in the most memorable way possible. In this type of article diagrams and graphs often serve his purpose well by embodying his message in an easily remembered picture. The hints on presentation to be given here are concerned with the second type of article. Its aim is to record a discovery in such a way that the facts and the inferences drawn from them can be examined with precision from every viewpoint and withstand all reasonable criticism of their validity.

Quantitative observations are made by either enumeration or measurement. Consequently even before he starts to enumerate or measure—let alone present his numerical results—an investigator would be wise to consider carefully whether valid or even credible quantitative observations can be made. For instance, the effect of treatment on relieving pain, or diminishing nasal "stuffiness," or improving joint mobility is a type of study that is often carried out. But to obtain valid numerical expressions of the effect in such cases may be the most difficult part of the whole investigation. In other words, enumeration and measurement may be required for a comparison yet in the absence of the correct criteria give a meaningless result.

One of the commonest questions asked is, How much detail should I give in my numerical results? An investigator has perhaps measured the blood pressures of 100 patients, given them a hypotensive drug for three months, and measured their blood pressures again to see what benefit has come from the treatment. Should he give all the recordings made on both occasions? Or the mean (average) blood pressures alone? Or the mean plus some measure of dispersal such as the standard deviation? No fixed rule can be offered, but this question needs to be considered afresh in every case with the following idea in mind: the object is to present the observations in enough detail to allow the reader to examine critically the inferences drawn from them yet sufficiently summarily to bring out their meaning. The reader does not want either a profusion of numbers looking like a computer print-out or a stark total that has swallowed up all the details. Such data are often adequately summarised in a frequency distribution with mean and standard deviation. Too often they appear on the page in the form of a histogram which is impossible to read precisely.

When the time comes actually to set out the numerical results, an author would be well advised to check them against each other and go through the arithmetic again. This elementary advice is mentioned only because many readers would be amazed if they knew how often conscientious editors find simple errors of this kind in papers when preparing them for publication. Another point the author should note is whether he has confused two different categories, such as patients with organs. For example, "Out of 20 patients 18 eyes had a visual acuity of less than X" (but in how many patients?). Another error of this kind is a failure to assign observations to logically distinct categories. For instance, the ages of a series of patients are grouped as 20–25, 25–30, 30–35 years, etc, or blood pressures as 70–75, 75–80, 80–85 mm Hg. The correct categories for the ages are 20–24, 25–29, 30–34, because "24" means right to the end of 24 until the clock chimes and that person becomes 25. But I know from correspondence with authors that this idea, so evident to most people, is elusive to some and to a few remains for ever incomprehensible, even unto the perdition of publication.

Though slovenly authors sometimes omit the units from measurements if their nature is obvious, it is best always to include them. Blood pressure should not appear as 120/80, for example, without the units, mm Hg. The introduction of the Système Internationale for the expression of measurements means that, whatever units were used in carrying out the work reported upon, they should be translated into SI units for publication, so that either the work should be reported in SI units or the older units should be followed by the SI equivalent in parentheses. Here it is worth mentioning that μ is not a unit. It no longer means "micron"; this measure is now μm. The symbol simply means one millionth and it qualifies the actual units as in μg, μl, μs. The last of those is a reminder that the international symbol for seconds is not sec but s, in contrast to what most authors still believe, and for hour it is not hr but h. Incidentally no symbol has a plural form: 10 mg, for example, does not have an s.

In the construction of tables and figures—that is, diagrams—for the presentation of numerical data the following passage from Bradford Hill[1] is worth bearing in mind:

"Graphs should always be regarded as subsidiary aids to the intelligence and *not* as the evidence of associations or trends. That evidence must be largely drawn from the statistical tables themselves. It follows that graphs are an unsatisfactory *substitute* for statistical tables."

When preparing a table an author should carefully consider its exact purpose, for a table provides an analysis of the data. It always classifies data, often summarises them, and should present them in a logical arrangement that allows a reader to make comparisons or draw inferences from them easily. In a scientific paper the author should always give a table a caption stating its contents, and then explain the contents more fully in the text. Needless to say, figures in tables should be added up correctly and agree with those given in the text. The table itself should usually have three horizontal and no vertical lines. The first and third horizontal lines mark the top and bottom of the table, while the second separates the headings within the table from the columns below them. Sometimes additional short horizontal lines come between the first and second to separate off subordinate headings over the columns. Patients should be identified by numbers, never by initials, in tables (and text) lest their identification lead to a serious breach of confidentiality.

In the preparation of figures—that is, curves of various kinds, histograms, dot diagrams, and so on—the aim is to bring out clearly the relationships between variables, often how one variable changes with another. Simplicity in illustrating this relationship will win the busy reader's attention. When checking the drawing of the figures it is as well to check also that abbreviations and symbols are identical with those in the text and in the approved international form if there is one. Very few journals nowadays redraw the diagrams sent in for publication, so that authors must take the whole responsibility for their clarity and legibility on the page. Collaboration with a skilled illustrator may be helpful.[2]

In presenting statistical results authors need to bear in mind that the standard deviation (SD) and the standard error of the mean (SEM) have different purposes. The SD is a measure of the dispersion of the things measured. The SEM describes the precision of a sample mean as an estimate of the population mean. Too often the SEM is reported when the SD is needed, because the SEM is smaller and thus seems to give a greater air of precision to the mean. An unfortunate convention has grown up of denoting the SD and SEM by the symbol $\pm$ tacked on to the mean, often without any explanation from the author of which expression his

204

symbol denotes. He writes, for example, $2 \cdot 5 \pm 1 \cdot 2$. Is $1 \cdot 2$ the SD or the SEM? He must tell his readers which. A better convention is to write: mean $2 \cdot 5$, SD (or SEM) $1 \cdot 2$. Another type of confusion lies in such expressions as: SD (or SEM) $= \pm 1.2$. The SD and SEM are positive quantities that can be added to or subtracted from the mean. They are not negative numbers, as that expression implies they may be.

If numerical data are presented to allow a comparison of some sort to be made, a statistical test of the significance of one or more differences between them is nearly always advisable. For instance, a paper showed that 43 patients out of 50 (86%) improved on treatment A while only 20 out of 30 (67%) improved on treatment B. The authors simply left it at that, but a χ^2 test with Yates's correction shows that the difference is not significant at the 5% level. The authors ought to have carried out this or a similar test because their results cannot be reliably interpreted without it. But, if they had, they would have then had the problem of telling their readers what practical inference to draw from it. Some might take the risk of saying that though the difference is not significant at the 5% level it nevertheless indicates a trend that has a bearing on clinical practice. Some would not take that risk because even a 5% level is not at all stringent. Nor is it justifiable simply to add some more cases in the hope of getting a definite answer. Authors who want to publish data that have not reached a conventional and quite low level of statistical significance need to exercise the greatest care in drawing conclusions from them and should usually seek the guidance of an expert statistician.

But even an expert statistician may fail to give the right kind of help if he is consulted too late or advised inadequately. For example, a team of investigators have produced a mass of numerical data and they ask a statistician to make all sorts of comparisons between them. Perhaps he does 20 tests and only one of them is significant at the 5% level. On chance alone this is not unexpected (as he will probably point out), but the investigators use it in their paper, albeit with a slightly disconsolate air, to prove that X is a better tranquilliser than Y, at least for unmarried women with red hair, aged 30–32, whose occupation is personal assistant and whose water supply contains less than 1 ppm of magnesium.

A fallacy of a similar kind can lie in the production of a significant result from an intricate statistical analysis when a simple method applied to a straightforward comparison has failed to give one. It is true that the intricate method may have succeeded because it has made use of more information than the simple one and thereby allowed a more complete comparison. But its success may also be due to the fact that some of the information it uses has little or no importance in clinical practice.

Many observations made in clinical medicine are of necessity approximate in their measurement, variable from time to time, and responsive to the investigator's attitude and skill. The application to them of complex statistical methods can easily lead an investigator to draw conclusions that are more precise or refined than the data can properly bear. Two points are worth remembering here: it is far more difficult to make an exact observation than to do a simple statistical test; and statistical significance does not necessarily imply practical significance.

The difficulty of making an exact observation is matched in clinical practice by the difficulty of making a valid comparison. Statistical methods allow to a certain extent for the averaging out of differences, and in the selection of individuals to make up groups for comparison the use of tables of random numbers is now standard practice. But in reporting the results the investigator should state clearly the composition of his groups so that readers can judge their comparability. Thus it is far too casual merely to say that two groups of patients were comparable in all important respects. Among the attributes in which groups of patients are commonly required to show similarity are age, sex, and socio-economic class or occupation, together with many others in special circumstances, such as family history, personal history, previous exposure to an infection, inoculation state, severity of disease, type of pathological lesion, and prognosis. These attributes or whatever others are considered important to the outcome of the investigation should be clearly set out for the reader's inspection.

Though statistical analysis of clinical data is generally best restricted to simple methods, much ingenuity and subtlety may be needed in planning the investigation that is to provide the data for the analysis. Consequently before presenting the numerical results an investigator should describe the plan of research clearly, for besides setting the results in numerical form his task is to convey their full and exact meaning. The reader wants not merely numbers but the practical realities that they measure.

---

[1] Hill, A B. *Principles of medical statistics.* 9th ed. London: Lancet, 1971.
[2] Swinscow, T D V. Faulty illustration: a personal view. *J Audiovisual Media Med*, 1983; **6**: 105-6.

206

Write a paper

ALEX PATON

Don't believe people who tell you that writing is easy. Except for the fortunate few, writers are made, not born, and the fashioning is a painful process—a very private struggle between you and a blank sheet of paper. Fortunately for the medical author there are certain guidelines and plenty of advice, but the challenge remains. Doing the research or collecting case material is child's play compared with the moment of truth when you come to write up (or down) your results. But given that you have something worth saying— and too many papers seem to be written because someone other than the author thought it would be a good idea—get down to it, learn a few basic rules, and write—and write.

The structure

The writer of scientific and medical papers has the advantage of a ready-made scaffold on which to build. This is the IMRAD structure and corresponds with the questions (table) which Sir Austin Bradford Hill said an author should try to answer. If you wish you can start with the *Introduction* and work straight through, but you don't have to; sometimes it is easier to begin with *Results*, because this is the core around which the rest of the argument can be written. Most introductions need only a couple of paragraphs, at the most; they do not require a review of "the literature." *Materials* (or *Patients*) and *Methods* should also be short. You do not need to give details of common techniques, but if your work is based on a new method you must provide adequate details so that others can repeat it. This is not always done with sufficient care, and gives rise to a suspicion, no doubt entirely false, that the author does not want other people to verify his work. *Results* are results. One of the commonest faults is to introduce snippets of interpretation into this section; the proper place for them is in the discussion. The *Discussion* is always difficult. If you are stuck, begin by giving your results in the light of other people's findings, proceed to discuss their meaning, and end by stating how they alter or advance current ideas. If possible, indicate future lines of research.

Structure of an article (Imrad)

ABSTRACT

I ntroduction	Why did you start?
M ethod	What did you do?
R esults	What did you find?
A nd	
D iscussion	What does it mean?

There is no need to sum up or conclude at the end of the discussion. Most journals now print an abstract at the beginning of the paper, and this is often the only part that people read. Take as much trouble (or more) over composing the abstract as in writing the paper. It must contain the points that you wish to get across as factually as possible, and should not be more than 250 words.

The practice

I write it all out in long hand just as it comes, though other people may prefer the typewriter or Dictaphone. Having summoned up the courage to begin, you cannot at this stage get tied up over niceties of style or meaning and you must keep on writing. It may help to prepare notes of the points you wish to make, and to pepper the pages of the manuscript with headings so as to maintain direction.

Next I type out (or preferably have typed, as I am a two-finger man) the written draft with wide spacing all round, including the margins. If you think that your first attempt was sheer hell and that the worst is over, you are in for a shock, for it is now that the hard work begins. You will find that the manuscript has to be corrected and corrected again, so that it ends up almost unreadable. I spend hours worrying about choice of words and the sequence of ideas, and often have to cut the script up, to cut out sentences and paragraphs and shuffle them around. They can then be pasted back in their new position on another sheet of paper.

Having got as far as possible, you have the manuscript retyped and put it aside to mature. Unless you are working to a deadline (a useful discipline) there is no point in hurrying, however ambitious you are to see your name in print. Editors of medical journals have little sense of urgency and your claim to have discovered a cure for ingrowing toenail is unlikely to impress. I give my paper to someone else to read, someone who will tell me the truth (often unpleasant when it applies to my masterpiece) and maybe give some practical help. I would like to see one or two people in each department or hospital prepared to read and criticise papers, not for the scientific content (that is a matter for colleagues in the same field) but from the viewpoint of the general reader. It might then be possible to dispense with editors.

After a month or so you will begin to feel an irresistible urge to have another look at the paper. You will hardly recognise it and can see at once its many shortcomings. It has to be rewritten once more, but this time the task is easier and there are fewer hang ups. It is now essential to give the revised draft to a secretary who knows the style of the journal to which you are submitting the paper, and she may then type the final or, if you are less confident, the penultimate copy. Note that there have been four, possibly five, drafts; it is not usually possible to get away with fewer.

The package

I hope editors are human enough to be favourably influenced by a nicely presented paper. You don't necessarily need to start writing with a journal in mind, but by the second or third draft you should know where it is to be submitted. You have studied the style of that particular journal, the length of its articles (particularly important in these days of economy), and its notice to contributors. Unfortunately the variety of different styles and instructions is enough to put off the most dedicated author, and I am an active campaigner for uniformity in matters such as references, but it is bad manners to send off a paper to a journal you haven't bothered to look at.

The final copy of the manuscript must have double spacing, wide margins (for subediting), and be typed on one side of the paper only. Send three clean copies with the minimum of penned alterations—dogeared copies that have obviously been the rounds are unlikely to be accepted. The first (and separate) page should contain the title, together with the names of the authors, their degrees and appointments, and the name and address of the author to whom correspondence is to be sent. It is often useful (sometimes essential) to provide a "short title." The abstract follows on the next separate page, and then the text itself. A short covering letter, not a full length apologia, should be signed by all the authors.

The title is very important, both to catch the eye of the reader and for indexing. Many authors seem to think that titles must be long, dull, and "scientific," instead of trying to follow the example of writers like Richard Asher or the anonymous composers of newspaper headlines.

If you are reporting large numbers of patients or experiments, which are split into groups, make sure they tally in text and tables. A reader who finds that figures don't add up rapidly loses interest. Tables should be typed separately from the rest of the text. It is difficult to say anything succinct about illustrations since journals vary in their practice, but if you send photographs label them on the back in pencil with author's name, short title, and "TOP" with an arrow. Photographs have a nasty habit of getting separated from manuscripts in editorial offices or of being printed upside down. Be particularly obsessional about references—it pays to have a librarian or secretary who likes chocolates. Be sparing over acknowledgments, but avoid making enemies for life by leaving out genuine helpers.

The style

I have left to the last what is for the amateur undoubtedly the most difficult part of writing—style. The first (and rarest) quality is brevity: short words, short sentences. Why is it that intelligent people (among whom I include doctors) become imbued with verbosity the moment they put pen to paper? A staccato style must be avoided, though, and the best way to "pace" the writing is to read it aloud. Need I emphasise to a scientific audience the importance of accuracy and the correct word? We all use words not only without knowing their true meaning but also without appreciating their shades of meaning. When you write that "your results revealed . . ." do you really mean that they were "made known by divine or supernatural agency" (*OED*)? It is a valuable exercise to make up sentences in which a key word—for example, the verb—is missing and to see how many alternatives can be used and which are the most appropriate.

Try to avoid vogue words like the plague (and clichés like that) Philip Howard, whose style is worth studying, wrote a series in *The Times* in which he pointed out how the meaning of such words eventually becomes completely distorted by popular usage, words such as parameter, charisma, consensus, obscene, interface. As for "situation" its present vogue is really becoming something of a "headache situation," as I have heard a difficult problem described. There are clichés confined to medicine which make the hackles rise: "disease process," "the patient went rapidly downhill," "the patient presented to hospital."

Watch out too for the circumlocution, the round about talk, the gobbledegook beloved of civil servants and sociologists. Much of the "noise" can be removed altogether or replaced by a single word. In the fullness of time (cliché) we shall be introducing literary audit (vogue word) for medical writers, and one of the more difficult tasks (for specialist registration) will be to précis circulars from the DHSS. You should develop a special alarm system for in-words, such as "red in colour," "moment in time," and for un-words—"it is not unusual," "it is not unexpected." Finally, try to use short, concrete, Anglo-Saxon rather than Romance words, which tend to be long, abstract, and imprecise. Dr Johnson, as always, provides the apposite example, which we imperfect writers might well display prominently in our studies: "It possesses insufficient vitality to preserve it from putrefaction" can be rendered both simply and devastatingly, "It has not wit enough to keep it sweet."

There are many books and articles giving guidance to the writer and I have prepared a list of my favourites. In them you will find not only good advice but so many warnings of the pitfalls that all but the most daring will be put off. Don't forget that much can be absorbed with pleasure from one's everyday reading. But in the final analysis nothing succeeds like repeatedly doing a job yourself and, to leave you with a few crumbs of comfort, I pass on the words of a respected journalist friend who, when asked how he managed to write with such ease, replied: "The first million words were the worst."

Further reading

Allbutt, T C. *Notes on the composition of scientific papers*. London: Macmillan, 1925.
Apley, J. *Br Med J* 1976; i: 999.
Asher, R. *Richard Asher talking sense*. London: Pitman, 1972.
BBC. *Words*. London: BBC Publications, 1975.
Booth, V. *Writing a scientific paper*. Colnbrook: Koch-Light Laboratories, 1971.
Fowler, H W. *A dictionary of modern English usage*, 2nd ed. Oxford: Clarendon Press, 1965.
Gowers, E. *The complete plain words*. Harmondsworth: Penguin, 1962.
Hawkins, C F. *Speaking and writing in medicine*. Springfield: Charles C Thomas, 1967.
Kohn, A. *Principles and methods of obscurantism, New Scientist*, 29 January, 1970.
Lancet. *Writing for the Lancet*. London: Lancet office, undated.
Lock, S. *Thorne's better medical writing*, 2nd ed. Tunbridge Wells: Pitman, 1977.
O'Connor, M, and Woodford, F P. *Writing scientific papers in English*. Amsterdam: Associated Scientific Publishers, 1975.
Roget, P M. *Thesaurus*. London: Longman, 1962.
Wilson, G. *Bulletin of the Ministry of Health and Public Health Laboratory Service*, 1965; **24**: 280.

Attract the reader

J W HOWIE

Nobody compels a writer to write or a reader to read. A writer who wishes his writing to be read must be fully and sharply aware that it is up to him first to attract and then to hold the reader. The first need is to write a good title.

Unless the title interests me, I go no further. The content must be clearly indicated, but the form of the words is also important. A highly unappealing title is any one which has the weak schoolboy-essay form: "The (whatever it is) followed by of"—for example, "The incidence and sources of salmonellas in chickens" will not attract readers, who might respond to "How chickens acquire salmonellas." The short title with an active, brisk flavour and a clear indication of what is in the article makes a good start to winning a reader.

The names and addresses of the authors also matter. Well-known authorities writing from departments of good repute enjoy an advantage—grossly unfair, of course—over unknowns. Journals that do not give authors' names and the titles of their papers in an obvious place—that is, on the front or back cover page—do their contributors a poor service. With so many journals to be looked at in order to keep up to date, the busy reader is very apt to skip those which hide their contents page among advertisements.

Need for an informative summary

After the title, I look at the summary; so the best place for this is just after the title and authors' names. If the summary is informative, I am encouraged. If it is merely indicative, I am discouraged. An example of an indicative, weak summary would be something of this sort: "An extensive survey of chickens in various situations has been made to ascertain the incidence and points of origin of salmonellas. The results show where infection has been acquired and point to the need for further research." This will deter any but the toughest readers. Waverers might be won by something stronger like this:

"Five thousand chickens were examined for salmonellas in 20 farms, three processing plants, and 100 shops. Infected feed containing fish meal on one farm was found to result in widespread contamination of birds from that farm and through them of clean birds as they passed through one processing plant. We conclude that efforts to produce clean poultry feed and to improve the hygiene of farms and processing plants will do more to control food poisoning than the numerous, currently popular but futile searches for human so-called carriers in shops, restaurants, and homes."

This essentially informative and controversial statement of conclusions will compel me to read further to see if the prima facie evidence is good enough. If it is, the case for further research along these lines needs neither argument nor statement.

Where is the evidence?

If the author and editor have done well by the reader, there will be an easily read section containing all the results and observations. Here there will be tables, graphs, histograms, or illustrations with just enough supporting text to guide the reader through the evidence from beginning to end; and there will be a statistical evaluation where this is necessary and relevant. There is no need to present the same evidence in graphic and in tabular form. The need is to choose which form most clearly and accurately gives the facts to the reader.

The evidence section is the real heart of any good scientific paper, and it is what the author should first assemble if he shares my view of what he is doing for his reader. If it satisfies his own critical judgment he should then write the informative summary in order to focus his mind on the essentials of his message. He will thus discover if he has indeed a worthwhile message to deliver and he will have given himself a clear picture of what is relevant and what is merely incidental to its presentation.

What is next?

If the evidence is good and the results are interesting, I next wish to know what the authors make of them. Where do they take us? So I turn to the discussion and, if it is convincing I shall next look at the introduction and review of previously published papers on the same subject. Involved discussions of a quasi-philosophical, theological, mystical, or autobiographical nature are not welcome. The discussion needs life and colour. A bit of controversy is good for interest, but it must not be manufactured or forced. It can readily be carried too far; and personality conflicts are out of place. A good discussion will make me read the introduction and review of the literature to see why the work was undertaken and if the paper is really advancing knowledge and understanding. Long preambles are not needed to justify undertaking a piece of investigation, and exhaustive bibliographies are exhausting. Authors have a duty to read other workers' papers and to study them exhaustively but they do not need to prove the extent of their virtue to ordinary readers of journals. Admittedly the matter is different if the reader is the examiner of a thesis; but this is not what we are considering here.

Lastly, if I am engaged in the authors' field of work, I small want to read their methods carefully and critically. Standard methods may be cited by reference, but new ones or modifications of established ones must be given in enough detail to allow interested persons to repeat them accurately. When I was responsible for honours students, I found it a good exercise for them to try to repeat new methods described in papers relevant to their studies. Almost always, the methods were either incompletely or inaccurately described and could be reproduced only after correspondence with their authors.

Discussion

Keeping up to date is a responsibility in which doctors often fail their patients. Of course, doctors are busy, but they are bad doctors if they stop reading about their subject. Writers must make their articles readable if they are to be read; and they must realise the competitive nature of their quest for readers. During my active professional life I necessarily read a great deal—at home, in trains and buses, in the laboratory and office; but I never read as much as some applicants for posts claimed that they did. Latterly, I read two weekly journals and two periodicals (I had better not say which) besides many manuscripts, reports, contents lists, abstracts, and reprints. I had to be highly selective, and I proceeded as described in this paper through title, summary, results, discussion, introduction, and review of the literature to methods and material in that order. If it helps writers of paper to have this account of one reader's approach I have reached my objective.

Referee a paper

D A PYKE

The arguments in favour of refereeing are:

(1) No editor can know his subject well enough to be an expert in all its aspects. This must certainly be true for a general medical journal, such as the *BMJ*, but I think it is true even for specialist journals. My particular interest is in diabetes. That sounds a narrow subject but there are five English language journals, each containing about 100 pages an issue, devoted entirely to this one subject. A quick look at the list of contents shows how varied are the papers: clinical, biochemical, pathological, statistical, and immunological. I do not know anyone who would claim to be an authority on all these aspects of diabetes. My view seems to be shared by the editors of *Diabetes* and *Diabetologia*; both these journals use referees.

(2) It takes a long time to establish a journal's reputation, but it may soon be lost if a few bad or hastily written papers or papers without proper acknowledgment of other work are published. It is the ease of making bad mistakes and their disastrous consequences that support the need for expert refereeing. (Referees make mistakes too—there is only one sure way of not publishing bad papers, which is not to publish any.)

(3) Most manuscripts can be improved by advice from referees. This may have nothing to do with grammar or style but may concern a reference that has been missed, a conclusion which is over bold, or a technique which needs description. The referee may see, in a way that an editor cannot, how a paper can be improved by amplifying or explaining part of the work, or that the paper would be better if deferred until more material has been collected or more experiments done.

The arguments against refereeing are:

(1) It causes delays. A paper can be killed by long delays in publication. Recently the process of publication has been speeded up in most of the more general medical and scientific journals

(*BMJ*, *Lancet*, *Nature*); refereeing takes time, so omit it. But referees can be prompt. In practice the time taken to referee a paper is only a fraction of the whole submission-to-publication time.

(2) Refereeing does not lead to the best selection of papers. A general editor can do just as well. My bias is against this, and I think poor selection of papers shows, at least to the expert reader.

I have set out some of the pros and cons of refereeing, but why must we come to any definite conclusion? Why not have variety? I am, in general, in favour of refereeing for medical journals but I am glad that there are some editors who never referee and some who break their own rules. The editor of *Nature* in 1953 cannot have needed a referee to advise him to accept that paper by Watson and Crick.*

If I were chairman of the journal committee of the BMA I would say to the editor: "I hope you will go on using referees but I also hope that you will use your own judgment, not merely on bad papers, which I am sure you can easily reject without advice, but also on good papers, whoever the authors may be. It may be easy to decide to accept a paper by Peter Medawar or Cyril Clarke, but you may also get a paper by someone you have never heard of which you like, and then I hope you will take it."

How to referee

(1) The editor must know what he wants from his referees: straight advice on whether to accept or reject or, in addition, criticism of the paper and, if so, in detail or only in outline?

The editor must choose his referees and they must have certain qualities—they must be reliable and punctual (unpunctuality is an incurable curse). An editor soon learns whose judgments cannot be trusted. My guess is that most referees tend to err on the side of recommending rejection and the editor may have put on a slight bias to compensate for this. On the other hand, a referee who recommends acceptance of a paper which is then demolished in correspondence should probably be dropped. A man may have been a good referee once but cease to be so because he does not keep up with his subject or takes on too many other commitments. He should be dropped.

Should the editor use one referee or more? If he uses a second referee, either simultaneously or after the first has reported and they disagree, what then? Use a third, or disregard them both? It is

---

* But even that great paper could have been improved! The first seven words of the famous last paragraph—"*It has not escaped our attention that* the specific pairing we have postulated immediately suggests . . ." are superfluous.

216

probably better, as a rule, to use only one referee but there will be exceptions. Indeed, a referee may himself suggest that the editor takes another opinion because he is unsure of his own judgment or is not familiar with the whole scope of the work being considered.

Should the editor transmit the referee's comments verbatim to the author? This question has been exercising the editor of the *New England Journal of Medicine*,[1] who fears that rude comments such as "waste of time" or "useless work" will offend the authors. Of course they will and there is no need to pass them on. All authors, whatever their protestations of indifference, are as sensitive as mothers at baby shows and just as protective. If an editor wants to reject a paper he can do so politely and, unless there is a special reason—for example, that the paper would be better in another journal—without giving a specific reason. Some may disagree with this advice on the ground that it lacks courage or is secretive, but I see no point in rubbing salt into the wounds of rejection—and another editor may accept the paper.

Should referees be named or anonymous? In theory referees should be named: the authors know whom they are dealing with and everything is open and acknowledged and the referee is restrained from indulging his whims and prejudices. I believe this is a facile argument and that referees will usually give better opinions if their identity is protected. They are spared the embarrassment, for example, of being seen to recommend rejection of a paper by a senior man or personal friend. Of course, the editor has to choose referees carefully when they are privileged by confidentiality and reject those with obvious bias, but that is part of good editing.

How to choose referees? In most subjects there are many experts in the country and from them good referees can soon be selected, but in some highly specialised fields an editor may have to reach across the world to find the right man.

If an editor rejects a paper he should be ready, if the author challenges him, to think again and perhaps consult another referee. A referee must accept that he is not the only adviser an editor may use and that he is giving an opinion, not making a decision.

The referee

Some simple rules:

(1) Don't lose the manuscript. A former chief of mine had a bad few hours before his secretary found a manuscript he had accidentally thrown away on the town rubbish tip. If you lose the author's only manuscript I advise immediate emigration.

(2) Be prompt. If you cannot read and comment on the manuscript (which does not usually take long) within two, or at most three, weeks return it at once. It doesn't take any longer to read the paper today than in a fortnight, and it won't go away if you put it in the bottom of the "in" tray.

(3) See what exact questions the editor is asking you. The editor of the *BMJ* asks specific questions about a paper: Is it original? Is it reliable? Is it clinically important? Is it suitable for the *BMJ* or would it be better in another journal?

(4) If in doubt add a bias in favour of recommending publication. A borderline paper published is not a sin, but a reasonable paper rejected is a shame. The temptation is for the referee to be superior and advise rejection. It should be resisted. The purpose of medical journals is to convey information, not to block it.

(5) Don't nitpick. There is a strong tendency of referees to find little faults. A referee may prefer one way of expressing results but if the author prefers another there may be no harm in that. The referee is not the author. In short, don't be bitchy. Your opinion may be confidential but write it in such a way that if it were published you might be embarrassed but not ashamed.

(6) Don't be overawed by the authors: famous men can do bad work and write bad papers. And papers from famous departments may be badly prepared and may not (or so one must suppose) even have been read by some of their illustrious authors.

(7) Don't ask silly questions of the author. Don't ask him if he has collected results which it is obvious he has not. If the absence of those results invalidates the paper advise rejection; if not keep quiet. Likewise don't suggest new work. You are judging this paper, not the next.

(8) Don't get bogged down in details. At the first reading take the paper at speed to get its general feel and then turn to points of technique or detail.

(9) If you have comments which you specially do not want the authors to see make that clear to the editor.

(10) Try to resist the temptation to advise acceptance of a paper merely because it makes frequent (and favourable) reference to your own work.

(11) Don't get in touch directly with the author, least of all by telephone. If referees are meant to be anonymous they should stay so.

Conclusions

I come back to a few points: referees usually improve a journal;

they should be anonymous, but they should write as if they were not; the editor should not usually give detailed reasons for rejecting a paper.

Finally, there are no absolute rules in this matter; variety is of the essence of progress, which is what medical publishing is for.

[1] Anonymous. *N Engl J Med* 1975; **293**: 1371.

Be your own subeditor

W F WHIMSTER

Articles pour into the medical journal offices. The editors try to judge them on their scientific value, but their task is difficult, since in very few does the scientific value shine out completely clearly. The language of most articles makes very hard reading—which does not endear them to the editors. The reading is made into work rather than pleasure by unnecessary words, inaccurate grammar, imprecise expressions, and abbreviations which distract the reader from the author's message. My aim is merely to make the message clear by removing the distractions from the writing, not to indulge in pedantry. At first some people are afraid that it may also remove their personal style and make it dull or flavourless but they are usually reassured by the results.

As a freelance subeditor or language supervisor, mainly for articles written by authors whose native language is not English, I have tried to identify the criteria I use to improve clarity. In fact, I find that I am looking to see whether the authors have applied the advice given by the other contributors.

I start by cutting away the verbiage until I can answer "Why did he start?" in the introduction (easily the worst done section); "What did he do?" in the methods section; "What did he find?" among the results; and "What does it mean?" in the discussion. Journal club members have many good opportunities to practise this—and will find themselves rejecting from their discussions many published articles because the answers are not there. I am aware, of course, that it is easy for a subeditor such as myself to change the meaning—I make my suggestions in pencil on the page so that the author or editor can erase them if they disagree with the new meaning.

I look at the grammar in a simple way—checking all verbs for their subjects; all pronouns for their nouns; all adjectives and adjectival clauses to see what noun they are telling me more about; all adverbs and adverbial clauses for the verbs they modify; and I examine every dull passive construction to see if it can be made active. I reject circumlocutions, woolly words, abbreviations (most readers cannot remember what they mean), and pomp, unless it is on purpose. The passage which follows shows many common examples of all of these failings, while the succeeding list shows how these infelicities may be improved. One has to be careful not to be carried away by this sort of thing, and it may need more than one attempt.

Introduction

Approximately 200 g of boro-lithium activated charcoal (BLAC) are needed *in order* to treat each severe case of *A phalloides* poisoning *at the present moment.* Ford *et al* (1975) *were of the same opinion* but they *anticipated* that deactivator coated charcoal would *be of assistance* to a wider *spectrum* of patients *at some future date.*

After treatment *commences* the urine becomes black *in colour comparatively* frequently and *a considerable proportion* of patients *demonstrate skin rashes due to the fact that BLAC* still contains impurities. *It may be noted* from *the literature* that *during the time* the rash lasts the serum charcoal *level* is *elevated in excess of* 20 mg/100 ml. *It is also probable* that the blood supply to the *lower limbs* is *significantly decreased relative* to the *upper limbs* in *females* on contraceptive therapy.

In this situation it seemed to the present writers that, *as already stated*, more *sophisticated* forms of charcoal therapy could be developed, and they *theorised* that experiments in which rats were *sacrificed following* charcoal dialysis would *reveal* new *data* about the interactions between charcoal and the new pomp-deactivator, Medipen.

This communication reports . . .

DISTRACTION	TYPE	HOW TO REMOVE IT
approximately	(3)	about
in order	(1)	(delete)
at the present moment	(1)	now
were of the same opinion	(1)	agreed
anticipated	(5)	suggested
be of assistance	(1)	help
spectrum	(3)	range
at some future data	(1)	(delete)
commences	(1)	starts, begins
in colour	(2)	(delete)
comparatively	(1)	(delete)
a considerable proportion	(1)	many
demonstrate	(5)	develop

DISTRACTION	TYPE	HOW TO REMOVE IT
skin rashes	(2)	rashes
due to the fact that	(1)	because
BLAC	(4)	boro-lithium activated charcoal
It may be noted	(1)	(delete)
the literature	(6)	previous work (refs)
during the time	(1)	while
level	(6)	concentration
elevated in excess of	(1)	above
It is also probable	(1)	probably
lower limbs	(1)	legs
significantly decreased relative	(3)	less than
upper limbs	(1)	arms
females	(1)	women
In this situation	(1)	(delete)
it seemed to the present writers	(1)	we thought
as already stated	(1)	(delete)
sophisticated	(5)	advanced
theorised	(7)	argued, suggested
sacrificed	(5)	killed
following	(1)	after
reveal	(5)	give
data	(1)	facts
This communication reports	(1)	in this paper, article

TYPES OF DISTRACTION

1 = pompous verbiage	22
2 = redundant word(s)	2
3 = technical word used out of its field	3
4 = irritating abbreviation	1
5 = wrong word	5
6 = imprecise	2
7 = unnecessary neologism	1
	36

I have illustrated these simple techniques because I am sure that each author, however eminent, should learn to do his "subediting" himself. Books often seem to get no subediting at all. As it is extremely difficult to do this objectively on one's own writing, the author should then enlist the help of a sympathetic colleague who also knows the rules. The colleague should go through it in front of the author, quizzing him on every point that is not absolutely clear. As this dialogue may become quite acrimonious, it is best for the colleague, however senior, to agree to a return match on his next paper. In this way differences in experience can be made constructive rather than destructive. Unintentional changes of meaning are avoided by this tête à tête verbal method, which is much better than the use of a remote subeditor. The latter can then get on with making the paper conform to the house style of the journal and with preparing the script for the printers. The remote subeditor is also spared the embarrassment of dissecting the verbiage only to find that the content is very small. With papers from non-English-speaking countries the subeditor will still have to spend some time in making the paper sound English to English ears, but this is a relatively minor task if the paper is well constructed in the first place.

As a pathologist I am naturally fascinated by the most elephantine example of any condition and conclude with a true one (though altered to disguise it) on which readers may spend a few happy minutes practising their subediting technique:

It is suffice to say that although substantial data has been presented demonstrating the antigenicity as well as the presence of tissue and species-specific antigens of prostatic tissue and other associated adnexal glands tissue of reproduction of the various species studied, the demonstration of the presence of tumour specific antibodies, or for that matter, circulating antibodies to prostatic tissue or secretions by the methods of precipitation and of passive haemagglutination in the sera of patients with benign or malignant diseases of the prostate and/or following cryosurgical prostatectomy has been, despite histologic and roentgenologic observations of the remission of distant metastates in cases of metastatic adenocarcinoma of the prostate (stage 3) following the cryosurgical treatment of the primary prostatic tumour, for the most part discouraging.

223

Edit a specialist journal

JOHN SWALES

It was really quite straightforward, I was assured, by the man who had preceded me as editor 30 years before. Papers were submitted and you read them. If they were good you accepted them, if they were not you did not: and that was clearly that. Unfortunately for the prospective editor of a specialist journal times have changed and he will find himself at the centre of a rather more complex operation. And so, when the ego-boosting invitation arrives, dear novitiate, it is as well to be prepared. You will, of course, have had some experience with scientific journals: you will have certainly been an author yourself; you will have acted as a referee; and you will have probably served on the editorial board. As a result you will probably have some ideas. If you have not you should probably decline the offer: you do not have the motivation to carry the task through. On the other hand, you may well suffer from some rather unrealistic ambitions. Perhaps you dream of a completely revamped journal stunning in appearance, each issue expectantly awaited by a rapidly increasing number of subscribers, the unchallenged leader in its field. It is as well to have some such praiseworthy but largely unattainable aims. My only advice would be to proceed with due caution and stealth. If not, most of your editorship will be spent trying to mitigate the errors of your first few months. Your failings will be displayed to a wide and attentive group of your peers. It may well be more worthwhile to take a fresh look at the content rather than appearance of your journal. There are some innovations which are certainly worth considering. Invited reviews, for instance, are more likely to be read, cited, and perhaps even enjoyed than original papers, and such reviews fulfil one of the major functions of your journal—which is to inform and stimulate.

The first thing to appreciate is that you are an amateur. Editing will be a part time task for you while you continue your clinical and academic work. You will, however, be supported by a fully professional staff at the journal editorial office. The senior staff will

224

have had many years' experience in producing journals and of dealing with the wilder eccentricities of editors and referees. If the editorial staff has no such experience then let someone else take on the editorship; the journal is heading for the rocks. Like most partnerships, that between an editorial office and an editor can become difficult if relationships are bad: that in turn is likely if roles are not defined. The staff at the editorial office (editorial managers, assistants, subeditors, etc) are responsible for the production of a journal from the manuscripts which you have selected and edited. Your job as an editor is to ensure that those manuscripts are of acceptable standard, both in form and content. You will therefore be responsible for seeing that the authors say what they have to say clearly and honestly. This may involve a good deal of work on the manuscript. The editorial office will then ensure that the printed version of the work will conform precisely to the style of the journal. This will involve a painstaking process of checking and "marking up" for the printer. These are professional procedures: if you as an amateur attempt them you may well cause more rather than less work for the editorial office (who may well be too patient and longsuffering to tell you). Your task should end therefore with a manuscript that reads as you wish it to read. Before the first paper leaves your hands you should know what is being done by means of an amicable discussion with the people involved. You should also determine the point at which a manuscript has been so altered by your efforts that the author should be asked to check and retype it before subediting is attempted. Setting up agreed procedures for dealing with these mundane matters is much more important than proceeding with your grand plan to change the covers of the journal to scarlet overprinted with the titles of the major articles in black. It is probably best to leave such things until a reasonable working relationship has been established between all concerned.

You will also inevitably be drawn into financial matters however much you protest that your role is purely editorial. To the outside world you are more closely identified with the journal than are the publishers. Here your lack of expertise may become even more painfully brought home to you, particularly if you have to participate in delicate negotiations between a learned society and a commercial publisher. I can offer only one guiding principle. By and large, the average specialist journal makes a healthy if not spectacular profit for its publisher. It is possible to test this, when a learned society owns the copyright, by putting the journal out to competitive tender. You will be surprised by the interest stimulated, an interest which is clearly not entirely altruistic. You may at this point decide that your own altruism is also limited and demand appropriate remuneration for your labours. You will certainly bear this in mind when asking for secretarial help.

These aspects of editorial work may not have crossed your mind before. As an author, however, you will have your own ideas about how manuscripts should be submitted and judged. This is a face you will present to your peers and you will yourself be judged just as much by this as by the appearance of the journal you edit. Whatever your feelings about the use of referees, as an editor of a specialist journal in the 1980s, you really have no choice if you intend your production to have scientific credibility. There is also little doubt that a minimum of two referees is required. Usually you will inherit an editorial process for seeking the opinion of referees. If not, you have a fundamental decision to make. Do you intend as editor to send papers to referees and reach your final decision unaided (except of course during unavoidable absence) or are you going to delegate some of your powers to assistant editors or members of the editorial board with expertise in different areas of your specialty? The decision you reach will depend to some degree on the number of papers you receive: more important, however, it will depend upon the breadth of interests represented by your journal. If it covers a wide area you may well not have the expertise to know who the reliable referees are: indeed you may well not understand the points at issue. It is not for you to resort to the more comfortable approach of the general medical journals "If the editors cannot understand it our readers will not understand it either and we should therefore reject it." Your journal is not only communicating reputable work as widely as possible. Very few people actually read what you publish. You and the subeditor will probably be the only people to read the journal from cover to cover. You have a duty to transmit to a select few and to act as an archive for valuable information which will provide a foundation for future work. You may therefore have to select a group of expert assistants from your editorial board who will seek the opinion of referees and advise you on what should be done with the manuscript. In this case your decision will probably be in most cases automatic or you may further delegate correspondence with the authors and the final decision to your assistants retaining for yourself only papers which lie in your own area. You will need to be fairly perspicacious in your choice of assistants: willingness is not always correlated with efficiency.

If you have tears to shed it will be shed over your dealings with the referees. To select a referee you have to form a shrewd idea of what the authors are trying to say by examining their manuscript briefly. You will then be able to decide on which of the sub-specialties the paper impinges. Some journals leave this to the editorial office. I believe this is quite wrong for two reasons. Firstly, you are asking referees to give a considerable amount of time to the task of assessing the manuscript. They are more likely to oblige a colleague whom they know than an editorial secretary. Secondly, the editorial office does not have the special knowledge to appreciate all the nuances in what may be a fine exercise of judgment. This is particularly true of work submitted to medical scientific journals where several discreet areas of expertise may be relevant. Let me put an imaginary example. An impressive paper may arrive reporting a startling increase in toenail uranium in patients with ischaemic heart disease. The authors conclude that uranium is a major risk factor. You send the paper to a leading international authority on the biology of uranium who reports that the methods are impeccable and the conclusions therefore of major importance. There are journals which would regard such a report as definitive: usually they belong to the small number of journals that attempt to cover all aspects of science from radioastronomy to molecular biology. When they venture into the medical word they tend to attach disproportionate importance to laboratory method. You however, dear editor, will be painting on a much broader canvas. Who are the people with ischaemic heart disease? Is it possible that their toenail uranium owes more to the fact that they are older and fatter, that they smoke and have quite different dietary habits from the authors' fellow scientists who served as controls in his study? You certainly need a uranium expert as referee: you will also need someone well versed in clinical research and epidemiology to advise you about confounding factors. You will thereby avoid propagating howlers which may help your position in the citation league as other publications refute the conclusions of the uranium paper but which will certainly not have helped the progress of clinical science. Your referees will therefore need to come from quite separate disciplines. This accounts for one of the two problems with referees which will dog your editorial career—discrepancies and delays. Your uranium and your epidemiological referees may well reach radically different conclusions about the adequacy of the manuscript. This does not mean that the refereeing process has failed. It simply means that you are (unconsciously perhaps) asking two quite different questions of different people. You may indeed indicate this in your covering letter to referees and reassure your epidemiologist that he does not have to worry about the validity of uranium measurement. This cannot be done by a subeditor or secretary inexperienced in the subject.

When reports are returned certain considerations have to be carefully weighed in reaching a judgment based on referees' views. Most journals use report forms to help in this task. The top sheet is for the eyes of the editor only and helps to concentrate the mind of the referee on the aspects of the paper which he is being asked to evaluate. Is the work scientifically acceptable?: how valuable a contribution is it? and how well is the work presented? A limited number of options can be presented from the hopeless to the outstanding. The top sheet also serves a secondary function in having cathartic value for the referee by inviting him to summarise his views and communicate any opinion which he does not wish the author to see. This section can be remarkably revealing. One of the first lessons which you will learn is that science at this level is not dispassionate.

On the second sheet the referee writes a report for the benefit of the authors. This also requires careful editorial study. Apart from the libellous, beware of statements which usurp your function such as "this paper would be acceptable if . . ." Authors have a habit of selecting the most optimistic assumptions upon which to act and you may find yourself having to justify an apparently anomalous decision which does not reflect the referees' views.

Whatever your personal views about the matter you are under an obligation to preserve at all costs the anonymity of referees. You are demanding enough of them without subjecting them to a potentially vituperative correspondence with wounded authors. The report sheet helps this by revealing only what the referee wishes to reveal. Without it you may find that one of your assistants has unwittingly transcribed rather more than you wished from a personal letter sent by a referee. If the referee identifies himself on the second sheet unwittingly and you overlook this fact at least some of the blame is his.

The behaviour of your referees will span the complete spectrum of human potential from the obsessional to the anarchic, from meticulous to the delinquent. Some will refuse to use your report forms, some will continue the remarks to you as an editor in the report for the authors. Some will tell you that the work is acceptable or not and leave it at that or simply that they disbelieve everything a particular author writes. In most of these cases you will make a mental note (or programme your computer) to dispense with the services of that particular individual. The worst form of referees' behaviour, however, is manifested by delay. Your editorial office will, of course, monitor the progress of the manuscript and will send regular reminders to the referee according to a plan which you have designed. At the end of six weeks the referees will probably be requested to return the manuscript with or without a report. Soon you will suffer the recurrent nightmare of the referee who after a delay of two or even three months returns the manuscript with a curt note of apology and no report. It is difficult at first to believe that there are many reputable authorities who behave in this way but your term as an editor will prove a revealing experience. No man is a hero to his valet and some scientific referees are by no means cast in the heroic mould as far as their editors are concerned. You are then left with a manuscript with one (occasionally no) report and an author who is scanning his post each day in vain. To deal with this situation you will have at your right hand a group of rapidly acting reliable referees who will provide a report (when the situation is gently explained to them) within a few days. The reputation of your journal and yourself depends upon the goodwill and efforts of such scientific saints.

On rare occasions you may feel it is necessary to preserve the goodwill of your referees by not sending a paper out to referee at all. This is a serious decision and not to be undertaken lightly but most journals receive the occasional crackpot paper or work which is quite inappropriate. When your clinical journal receives a paper on steroid levels in an obscure marine mollusc you will not wish to send the work to a long suffering precious steroid referee who reports that the work is technically good only to find that you have rejected it on grounds which should have been evident to you in the first place.

Now that you have your reports you are confronted with the delicate task of communicating with the authors. Your words will be studied in minute detail. Indeed the authors will probably spend longer on dissecting out the subtle implications of what you write than you have spent on composing it. Your aim is to present the conclusion which you have reached and provide guidance for the authors. To achieve this you must be quite clear what your decision is. If you feel that the work is not suitable for your journal it should be declined with appropriate expressions of regret. It is best to avoid detailed reasons describing where you feel the authors have gone wrong. At the most perhaps you should refer to the referees' reports, which should normally be sent with your letter. There may be a great many criticisms of the work and if you list only a few you risk tempting the authors to resubmit a manuscript which meets these points. You then have to explain that there was more to your original decision than you stated or gracefully give way. Some authors hold the view that most editors will give way if pressed frequently enough with a revised manuscript. It is up to you to disprove this hypothesis.

If the paper is probably acceptable you have to decide how you want the authors to revise it to meet the criticisms presented by the referees and yourself. If the necessary changes are trivial it is a reasonable courtesy to point out and indicate that the work is in principle at least acceptable. Many editors do not accept this view and presumably in terror of the possibility that they might enter a binding commitment to publish invariably begin their conclusions with the statement "I regret that your paper is not therefore acceptable to us." They then proceed "If, however, you . . ." This risks anticlimax when the major suggestion is to replace a couple of commas with colons and divide page 9 into three paragraphs. Often, of course, more major changes may be necessary. Here your letter becomes quite critical. The referees will have listed points which may, if you are fortunate, overlap but which may be quite discrepant. On occasions statements may be made which you feel should be ignored. You have to guide the authors through this maze describing what they must do to provide an acceptable paper. In some cases you may have to leave the final decision open and dependent on whether the authors can provide further data which they may or may not have. "I am afraid we could not accept your paper therefore unless you can present values for toenail uranium in a properly matched population as detailed by referee 2." Occasionally you may suggest a more modest paper in the light of the referees' comments. "We would therefore be happy to reconsider a paper describing and validating your method of measuring toenail uranium."

It is reasonable to provide your referees with some return for their work by sending them a copy of the other referees report (unidentified of course) and a copy of your letter. This will also help to ensure that justice is seen to be done.

If you have left the door only slightly ajar a revised manuscript will almost inevitably appear on your desk. The authors will also provide you with a reply to the referees with a list of changes that they have carried out. Your task is to assess their case and if you think it justifiable send the paper again to the referees for a second opinion. Where the points at issue are minor this is unnecessary. To enter the refereeing cycle a second (or third) time round is to invite profoundly irritating delays. Your role is that of a judge, not a tennis umpire, who watches helplessly as author and referee send the ball to and fro across the court.

And then when you have finally decided that you have an acceptable manuscript you will read it from beginning to end carrying out your editorial task before handing it on to your editorial office. Your grand design for the journal may well by now have been forgotten in the face of the need for sustained detailed work and your personal popularity may suffer in some quarters but you should ultimately have some tangible justification for your endeavours. You will have learnt something of your specialty and a good deal more about your fellow human beings.

Survive as an editor

STEPHEN LOCK

Editors survive by accepting good articles. Obviously there's more to a general journal than the original articles, but I believe that, however good and important the other sections are, its quality must depend on the quality of the papers, originals, and medical practice articles. What is a good article? It's one that has a definite structure, makes its point, and then shuts up. Its English uses nouns and verbs and not adjectives and adverbs, while the scientific structure is crisp and each individual section does what it is supposed to and no more.

How do we get good articles? We believe we can do this only by refereeing, or peer review. We ask our referees four main questions. Is the article original? Is it scientifically reliable? Is it clinically important? And is it more suitable for a general journal, or a specialist journal?

In depending so heavily on refereeing the *BMJ* of course differs largely from its distinguished contemporary the *Lancet*. Its last editor, Ian Douglas-Wilson,[1] is on record as saying that it is opposed to peer review, because it is too slow, because it tends to be conservative and élitist, and because it may be bigoted.

Given that a prime function of the editor is to monitor and control his referees, none of these objections seems to me very serious. With respect, the point about delay is trivial, because, as a recent article in the *New England Journal of Medicine* has shown,[2] the average time lapse between having the original scientific idea and publication of the final article is four years—of which only some five months is spent on the editorial process. I think also, to use a pompous phrase, editors should have a "social conscience." Doctors have been taught to read anything they see in a medical journal with a great deal of scepticism: they recognise that a classical path to a synthesis is by thesis and antithesis, and regard articles as contributions to a debate. Not so the general public: journalists are always on the lookout for stories, and a misguided or even wrong article reported in the general press can do widespread harm. I believe that this is more likely if articles are not refereed.

Elitism is a charge I can't understand. I've looked élite up in the *Oxford Dictionary*, and it means the choice part—the flower—of society. Surely if what editors want is the best, and assessment achieves this, then peer review is a good thing? Finally, it's up to the editor to monitor his referees—to know their likes, dislikes, and prejudices. At the *BMJ* we do this by using many of our referees first to write drafts of unsigned leading articles and then we try them on assessing papers. Now many distinguished people fail to make adequate referees: sometimes they're too kind or uncritical, but more frequently they tend to base the criticism on an ideal article which is in their heads and not on paper. What the editor is doing is to ask them for the views on an actual article, and if he finds that he cannot train a potential referee to give him straight answers to straight questions, the best thing is for them to part, at least so far as assessing articles is concerned.

Even after articles have been refereed, however, the editor is left with too many for the space available, and has the unenviable task of choosing them for the "general" reader. Although traditionally at the *BMJ* at least two of the editorial staff have been concerned with this, I have always been worried lest we were too far removed from clinical practice. Hence recently we have started copying the practice of the *New England Journal of Medicine*, which has a "hanging committee." At the *BMJ* now once a fortnight two editors discuss articles with one or two outside consultants. All of us have read the articles and the referees' comments and together we manage to reduce a pile of about 30 articles potentially suitable for publication to 12 for definite acceptance. This system helps to pick out a good article by a new and unknown author, and to find when a distinguished one has produced a poor paper—often probably because he has not actually written it, or even read the final result.

Poor English

But using a refereeing system and even good subediting after the article has been accepted should not be the only way of achieving good articles. The 5000 or so articles we see at the *BMJ* every year are mostly dreadfully written, with numerous faults in English and overall construction. Many of these articles, of course, are published somewhere largely in the original form, because if the matter contained in them fulfils the other criteria the editor has not the time to translate them into decent prose, and it is the author who signs them. Unfortunately these articles are not fulfilling their purpose: they are largely being left unread because of their turgidity.

Writing is now where speaking in medicine was just after the second world war. At this time, the Medical Research Society and the Surgical Research Society got together and devised a set of rules: that nobody should read an article; that the length of each contribution was limited to ten minutes; and that only a limited number of slides should be shown. These simple rules have improved the standard of spoken communication enormously, and I believe that unless something similar is done very rapidly for the written word people will largely stop reading medical journals. One way of doing this is to have general courses on medical writing; even better, is to have small group seminars discussing individual papers to illustrate various points; and a third idea, which is fairly common in major units in the United States, is to have one's own rewrite person to do the final polishing. Even so, I believe it is important for people to know how to write a good article, so that they recognise a good article when they read one.

The wrong medium

One common error is that articles are written for the wrong medium. Editors constantly see articles that have been written for speaking, but are quite unsuitable for publishing; and they go to conferences where doctors read articles that are perfectly suitable for publishing but inappropriate for delivering to an audience. Clearly in both types of article the author must have a very clear idea of the aim: otherwise his audience is going to find it too simple or too high falutin. But there are great differences in the *structure* (table I)—principally because speaking is a slow and relatively

TABLE I—*Structure*

	Speaking	Writing
Introduction	40%	5–61%
Main methods and results	40%	40–60%
Discussion and methods	20%	30–45%

inefficient way of getting information across. One of the first rules the BBC teaches its radio correspondents is that they can get only one idea across every three minutes. So if the average paper at a conference lasts 15 minutes, and three minutes are spent in introducing himself and another three in summing up, the speaker has time only to put over three ideas. In the published paper, of course, there's no such restriction. But three minutes is an awfully

233

TABLE II—*Content*

	Speaking	Writing
Ideas	One per 3 minutes	Theoretically unlimited
Repetition	Considerable	Minimal
Padding	Considerable	None
Style	Conversational Short sentences	Formal
	Few references and acknowledgments	Required number of references and acknowledgments

long time for one idea and this affects the *contents* of the spoken article (table II); it means that the speaker must repeat himself and pad things out a lot. Speakers naturally use jargon and imprecise words—those awful terms such as situation, and marked, and involved—because by gesture and the context the audience knows what they mean. In the printed word editors frown on such imprecise solecisms. Finally, in speech there's an opportunity for gimmicks over the *delivery* (table III)—jokes, gestures, slides, and so on. By comparison the austerity of the printed page is like a mausoleum.

TABLE III—*Delivery*

	Speaking	Writing
Adaptability to audience	Maximal	Limited
Arresting introduction	Important	Not often possible
Jokes	Desirable	Usually unnecessary
Visual aids	A few relevant slides	Minimum of relevant tables or figures
Length	Finish early	Short as possible

Nevertheless, both types of communication will fail if they do not have an obvious message, put over clearly, and briefly. Say what you have to say, and then shut up.

[1] Douglas-Wilson, I. *Br Med J* 1974; iii: 326.
[2] Roland C G, Kirkpatrick R A. *N Engl J Med* 1975; **292**: 1273.

Improve a student medical journal

COLIN M BARRON

I was always interested in magazines. At the age of 7 I produced my first—a 14 page collection of jokes, drawings, and stories entitled *The Weekly World*, and later I hand-produced a number of comic magazines for my own amusement. It was quite natural, therefore, that I should become interested in student publications, and during my undergraduate days I became involved with several magazines, especially *Surgo* (Glasgow University's medical journal).

Initially I was just a cartoonist, then a writer, later the advertisement manager, and finally I did a two year stint as editor. During these two years we were able to improve the production standards of *Surgo* considerably by applying a number of principles derived from years of success and failure. I hope they may be of value to others.

Key principles

Let's start at the very beginning. You're the editor of a student magazine which looks like half a dozen sheets of lavatory paper stapled together; the layout is abysmal; the articles are boring; and no one will advertise in it. Worse still, no one reads it. Just how do you start improving it? The first key principle is enthusiasm, optimism, and a genuine desire for improvement. If you do not enjoy being editor and do not want to make every issue better than the last, then you are in the wrong job.

The next important principle is to have a working knowledge of printing because an editor who knows nothing about printing is like a surgeon who knows nothing about anatomy. A good introductory text is the *Ladybird Book of Printing* (seriously) and most public libraries stock a few advanced books on the subject.

Production team

Having worked up some enthusiasm for your job, you should then assemble your production team. Ideally this should consist of several experts, each skilled in one particular subject. At the very least you will need an advertisement manager and a finance manager. If you intend to have much artwork in your magazine, you would be advised to have a couple of resident artists plus a photographer. If you do not have any design sense yourself, one of the artists should serve as layout man and art editor.

It is also useful to include in your production team some interested people who can serve as general dogsbodies—writing book reviews and snippets, for example, making coffee, and, most important, coming up with ideas.

Once you have assembled your production team encourage them all to contribute to the magazine in some way. It is wrong, I've found, to be *too* democratic—in the end the editor must have the final say because an unchecked committee will spend hours arguing about what colour of staples to use.

Layout and design

A common failing of student magazines is layout and design. Student editors are often content to present articles as page after page of unbroken type. In fact, the most interesting article in the world becomes unreadable when presented in this way, so if you want people to read your magazine learn about layout.

Unfortunately few books have been written about this and much of the craft seems to have been passed down by word of mouth, but you can learn by studying professional magazines. The next time you're browsing through *TV Times* stop and look. Observe the way that text, illustration, heading and white space have been blended together to produce a page that is attractive, eye-catching, and easy to read. It is worth while building up a collection of professional magazines with good layout for occasional reference. If you are really stuck for a way to lay out a particular article then go ahead and copy the layout from a professional magazine, inch for inch. Articles may be copyright but layouts aren't.

One of the basic principles of layout is that text should be broken up into small, easy to read blocks. There are several ways of doing this. The simplest is using subheadings in bold type surrounded by the correct proportion of white space. As it is rather unlikely that the author's original subheadings will occur in the most aesthetically pleasing part of the page, you may have to move the heading. More commonly, you will have to write headings that didn't exist in the original manuscript—whatever you do, however, don't waste the design value of a subheading by leaving it sitting at the top of a column.

Drawings and illustrations

Almost every article looks better with some sort of illustration and you should remember that it is usually the picture that makes people stop at a particular page. If you use drawings, they should be done in pen and indian ink—not a ballpoint pen or felt tip because this looks unprofessional. A Rotring-type indian ink drawing instrument is a good investment at about £4, while half tone areas can be effected with self adhesive dots such as Letratone.

Drawings look better if produced larger than required and then scaled down to size, and you can save on costs by having this done at a photocopying agency. Many of the latest copying machines produce enlargements or reduction of artwork whose quality is similar to bromide prints but at a fraction of the cost. Any photographs should be 35 mm black and white prints.

Avoid the temptation to cutout graphics from professional magazines for use in your own—as well as being a breach of copyright it is a rather obvious ploy. One student journal that I saw had to call its news page "Talking Shop" so that it could use a graphic from *World Medicine*.

A two column format is reckoned to be easiest to read, but if you use a lot of illustrations three (or more) columns allow a more flexible layout.

Cover design

I have singled out the cover for special mention because it is an area of graphic design that is often botched up in student publications. This is a pity because it is the most important page in your journal. Think how many times you have picked a magazine from the news stands because of an eye-catching cover.

The rules of cover design are quite simple and in the figure I have indicated the correct way to lay out a cover, and some of the common errors.

Your title logo should be set in a simple, easy to read, bold typeface and should occupy the greatest vertical height possible. Avoid hand drawn lettering—this never looks as good as Letraset, and the latter is cheap enough (for a limited amount of lettering) that there is really no excuse for not using it. Do not be tempted to use some of the over elaborate typefaces—medieval and futuristic styles look ridiculous on the cover of a medical journal, and

Common Errors in Cover Design

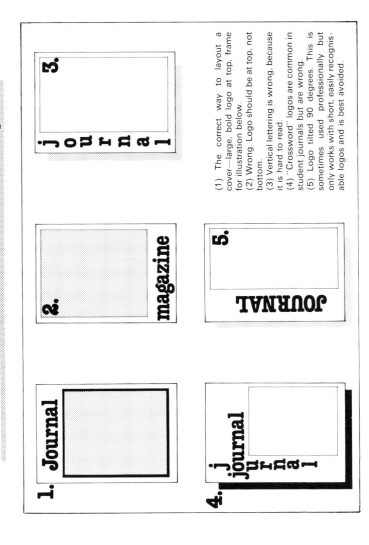

1. Journal

2. magazine

3. journal

4. journal

5. JOURNAL

(1) The correct way to layout a cover—large, bold logo at top, frame for illustration below.
(2) Wrong. Logo should be at top, not bottom.
(3) Vertical lettering is wrong, because it is hard to read.
(4) "Crossword" logos are common in student journals but are wrong.
(5) Logo tilted 90 degrees. This is sometimes used professionally but only works with short, easily recognisable logos and is best avoided.

remember that the simplest typeface is usually best. I would recommend Letraset's American Typewriter range of faces as, over the years, I have found them to be extremely versatile.

Advertisement manager

The advertisement manager is the unsung hero of the production team—without his efforts the whole show would not be possible. Regrettably, it is not a popular job and this is because people imagine that it involves many hours of letter writing, often with little result. But the job can be rewarding and fruitful and drudgery can be kept to a minimum if the right techniques are used. Letter writing can be dispensed with for selling advertising space, and the telephone used instead. The telephone is the most efficient way of selling advertising space—in our experience it has a success rate of over 50% as compared to 10% for letters.

When you are on the phone, try to put yourself in the shoes of the man on the other end of the line. What information would convince him that it would be a good idea to take an ad? The readership, for example. If a few copies of your magazine lie about hospital reading rooms then you would be justified in saying that your magazine is "widely read by doctors."

You should always try to present your magazine as favourably as possible, even if you do have to exaggerate somewhat, and if your magazine is still of poor quality then you should try to avoid showing a copy; you can do this if you sell space by phone. Advertisers are more interested in taking space if their product is in some way connected with features in the magazine. If you have a motoring section, for example, dealers will probably be delighted to take ads if you ask them to supply road test cars. If there is an annual ball coming up soon, try to get a clothes-hire service to advertise, and if you've got a book review section you should have little difficulty in attracting medical publishers.

Getting articles

The main complaint of student editors is that no one will write articles. There are several ways of getting round this problem. First of all, get as many regular features as possible. If someone writes a particularly good piece for one issue then make it into a regular feature. Regular features, once established, almost seem to write themselves and the editor need only send timely reminders as the copydate approaches. These regular features should be put on the same page on each issue to make them easier to find. If you're trying to get anyone to write for your magazine it is better to give them a subject or a title. A man who is asked to write about anything usually ends up writing about nothing.

Another problem is contributors who do not produce their articles on time. If this happens often it is a good idea to produce the article by interviewing the potential author and recording the conversation on tape. This can then be written up either as a formal interview or as an article with a few quotations. Most articles will need to be rewritten to some extent, to make them more palatable because the average contributor will be inexperienced. Even if you shirk rewriting the entire article, it is often worth rewriting the opening paragraph—as with other activities, the opening line is important and a better one can often be found a few lines further on. The title is important, too, and, in my opinion, it should be eye catching rather than just informative.

Finally, the last golden rule is perseverance. Even if you have early failures, it is important to keep trying. What I have described so far is the 1% inspiration. It is up to the student editor to provide the 99% perspiration.

Write a single-author book

G C COOK

Until relatively recently most scientific and medical texts were single-author works; those of Bacon, Darwin, Wallace, and Huxley are some examples. Most texts in the latter years of the nineteenth and the earlier years of the twentieth century were similarly written by one individual—for example, *Manson's Tropical Diseases: A Manual of the Diseases of Warm Climates* (1898). Such works have certain clear advantages: they express the personal viewpoints of the author, there is no danger of disparate and contrary views from different contributors, they do not consist of a composite accumulation of essays of differing styles with varying degrees of under- and overlapping, and the speed of production of the manuscript is in the hands of one individual. Above all, however, the great advantage is one of *balance*—something rarely achieved in a multiauthor work. A single-author book is therefore a personal work based on individual thoughts and research in much the same way as is an MD thesis. As well as being of contemporary value—that is, in gathering thoughts, ideas, facts and references from diverse sources—it might also be a record for which posterity will (hopefully) be grateful. Why has there been a steady and relentless increase in the numbers of authors, and also editors, in recent years? Clearly many factors are involved: increasing specialisation in medicine and science is obviously important; the time factor has become more critical as the pace and possibly the stresses of life have increased, and leisure time is at a premium.

Why undertake it, and have I got the time?

There must be a very good reason for embarking on this enormous task and it must never be undertaken lightly. The reason for writing must be compelling. There has been a vast proliferation of medical and scientific texts in the Western world over the past few decades; most of them are duplications of other works and they do not justify the amount of time spent on them.

Sometimes the major motive is the advertisement of the author's identity. Therefore, it must be original, preferably unique, and not just another book. It may be a record of original thoughts and new ideas. It might be an up to date systematic text preferably in an area not previously covered. It might be primarily a reference work—an accumulation of facts from the vast and diffuse literature in that particular field. Thorough justification must thus be forthcoming before the massive task is decided on. Writing will take up time normally used for patient care and teaching; however, it is research time which is likely to be eroded most of all. Adequate facilities, including a good library which covers the appropriate area, and a clear deadline for completion of the manuscript are essential. So time consuming is this venture that a stable marriage and tolerant children are perhaps the most important prerequisites.

How to start

When once the decision has been taken, a suitable publisher must be found—that is, if the work has not already been commissioned or requested. Only in rare circumstances should a book be written before a satisfactory publisher has been found and the contract duly signed; finding a publisher in retrospect can be a soul destroying business. It is well worth while to visit the general editor before starting the work and to keep closely in touch as writing proceeds. A satisfactory title which is short, precise, gives an accurate indication of the content, and which will enhance the selling power of the finished product is of great importance. It is also important to decide at whom the book is aimed—undergraduates or postgraduates, or is it primarily a reference work? Who will buy it? Individuals or libraries, and in which part(s) of the world will it be most relevant? A skeleton plan outlining a list of chapter headings is necessary; this can always be altered as writing proceeds, and inevitably will be as new ideas come to the fore. A system of numbering sections, chapters, and the subdivisions of chapters should be agreed with the publisher and strictly adhered to throughout. Preferably, a sample chapter should be written. The length can rarely be decided on before writing has started, but the manuscript must be as concise as possible. To most of us "x" thousand words means very little. Figures and tables might be included and they should be accumulated as the work progresses; they should be of the highest possible quality, especially clinical photographs, radiographs, etc. It must be a complete work in its area of expertise: a book which does not cover all that it sets out to do will inevitably be reviewed badly. As with original papers, reviews, and above all theses, the most difficult task is to put pen to paper; when once that is achieved the work will hopefully "snowball."

Preparation of the manuscript

It is essential that the publisher's style, and especially the form of references, is used from the outset, otherwise much time will be wasted. There can be no concrete advice on the best way to proceed with writing: to start at page one and proceed right through to the end, or to keep a section or several chapters running at the same time. Personally I find the latter approach gives rise to a more even balance. A precise style is essential. Is it primarily a reference work or a monograph incorporating new and original viewpoints? As many new and if possible original ideas should in any case be included. Attempt to expose unexplored areas, and throw out ideas for research projects if at all possible. Recent review articles should be combed with care, especially those from the better scientific and medical journals; they give valuable ideas regarding up to date references in the literature. How many references to include will vary enormously.

An easily intelligible free hand, and a secretary who can read it with ease, are enormous advantages. It is wise to get completed chapters (in draft) typed and corrected while they are still fresh in the mind. One draft followed by the final should be aimed at— otherwise expense becomes a real problem; an additional draft for some chapters will, however, sometimes be necessary. Use the blue pencil liberally; absolute accuracy is what matters in the final work. The completed top copy must be very carefully corrected, and that applies especially to the references to published work. Page numbering is best undertaken with an automatic numbering machine. Always keep a copy of the entire work to safeguard against loss or fire; what a "disaster" if the only copy goes up in flames.

When is the most suitable time to write? Isolation from the "hurly burly" of everyday life is the ideal. For example, I wrote a text on *Tropical gastroenterology* (Oxford University Press) while working in Papua New Guinea; the air conditioned medical library at the university medical campus in Port Moresby proved an ideal environment. But few find that relative luxury. It is essential to reserve specific periods—early mornings, evenings, weekends, etc. With patient care and teaching, let alone research, life becomes very full. Self-discipline and rigidity is required, otherwise the deadline will rapidly approach and much will still need to be done.

Finishing touches

The foreword and acknowledgments will usually be written as the work reaches its conclusion. The publisher will require some notes for the dust cover; do not be afraid to sell yourself. And then there is the index. How important that is, and how many books have been ruined by an inadequate index. Reviewers are on to a bad index like a ton of bricks. It should always be composed by the author for he or she knows and has a feel for the work. It is a long and tedious chore which comes when all seems to be over, but it is extemely important that it is well done. If it is a reference work the index should be long and detailed. Always have important references printed in a heavy typeface. A system using index cards is vitally important, and cross indexing is essential.

Ultimately the page proofs arrive. This is the last time you will see the work before it is published. Although it is, of course, essential to keep the corrections to a minimum, scientific accuracy is of paramount importance; reviewers and posterity will pounce on mistakes, however minor they are. Accuracy of references to published work is extremely important; that applies particularly if the book is relevant to Third World countries where it is often necessary to send off to libraries in the West, at considerable expense, for photocopies of original work.

The task completed

Eventually, after a never ending latent period between submission of the manuscript and arrival of the book, the project seems to be complete. One hopes that the proof errors have all been corrected, and the more obsessional author will meticulously check that that is so. Now, the reviews are eagerly awaited and the book swims or sinks depending on them.

After the publisher has filled all relevant libraries throughout the world with hardback versions, will a paperback edition be produced? The English Language Book Society (ELBS) may do this. Many factors determine whether this happens, and of course sales are greatly boosted by a cheap edition. Do not expect to "make a mint," for apart from exceptional cases—for example, a widely selling paperback—you will not. This is essentially a labour of love. And now prepare for the next edition—hopefully in some five to ten years' time. All relevant literature should be carefully recorded in a card index system. If available, a word processor is of incalculable value. The task is endless but, hopefully, worth while.

244

Deal with a publisher

H A F DUDLEY

The best advice that one can give to a potential author is "Don't." Books are highly labour intensive. If your work doesn't succeed there is the misery of having put in a great deal of effort without any reward; if it does there is the possibility of being on the treadmill of successive editions when other interests or imperatives are crowding in. And yet, and yet . . . a book is a creation and men and women seem driven by a creative urge. A book may be a succes d'estime and so put an author that much higher up in the pecking order. Finally, like all speculators we feel that *our* book will be a financial winner so that, like the writer of *Kennedy's Latin Grammar*, one may retire in early life to the Azores to live ever afterwards on the proceeds. So the urge persists and probably in this respect I am wasting my time. Even with negative and cautious advice from the experienced such as myself the new author in particular will rush in, forgetting as he does so that there is a professional side to books just as there is his medical work.

Now I have nothing much against publishers (and indeed they have grounds for having more against me), but I have to say that in the past they have not done a great deal to help medical authors either to make the best of their limited time and resources or to avoid the contractual pitfalls which can deprive individuals of their just rewards. Thus, the inexperienced author may either approach a publisher in innocence and ignorance or, if he is an attractive proposition, be approached, and negotiations in relation to both organisation and renumeration go a long way and even become irreversible before the author has really got himself experienced enough or advised enough to handle the matter effectively. So, do not get too deeply involved at an early stage. If possible have your whole book, an extended outline, or a draft chapter available before going to a publisher at all. Research the market through your friends and colleagues so that you can tell a publisher what his likely sales could be. Note in parentheses that a publisher works for profit and prices a book by dividing the estimated sales by costs to give a unit cost and adding the appropriate (have I chosen the right word?) margin. He worries about the "bottom line" of profitability and has to work on a gut feeling of what unit price the market will stand. When you finally see—if you get that far—what your slim volume will cost on the bookstall and experience a revulsion at its expense, remember these complexities. But I am getting ahead of myself. If the publisher does not like what you have to offer consider whether his criticisms are valid—there is more than an outside chance they may be. If they are, redraft and try again. If not, take your work elsewhere; publishers are for authors however much they may imply the reverse.

Having reached an agreement in principle the next stage is to produce the work if this has not already been done and to negotiate a contract. In both be realistic (I never have been and it has caused me and my publishers more angst than I would care to estimate). As to the writing, deadlines have got to be set either for your own work or that of collaborators. Allow one and a half times the most liberal estimate and try to beat it. This is not the place to give advice on writing techniques, which vary enormously and on which measureless secondary ink has been spilt. As to negotiating, remember that the publisher does have a living to make, a production schedule to draw up, and a financial risk to undergo. Remember further that he knows that your commitment to a book is not primarily financial and therefore that by comparison with a professional author you are not likely to try and go for very high rewards.

Most publishers' contracts now have many uniform features but they do differ enough to bear minute examination. My experience and that of others is that your solicitor (lawyer in Scotland) who has handled your house conveyancing and the tiff with the neighbours with expertise and despatch is not likely to have the right information or experience to deal with a contract about a book. What is more, he may very well not know he does not know and thus from his ignorance give bad advice. The alternatives are two: an agent, or join the Society of Authors. Agents, though real hardened experts, extract a considerable slice of the cake and are only really to be recommended to those who intend to make a considerable living from writing. I find that most reputable agents advise a medical writer against employing them. However, you may have an agent friend who will be prepared to help and if so hang on his every word. The Society of Author's is a distinguished protection group (and also a bona fide trade union) now a hundred years old. It was created expressly to look after authors and though most publishers like to deny that protection of any kind is needed, the publishing jungle remains a thick one with a few man traps for the unwary and the occasional author eater around. Though the Society's Medical Writers Group has only been in existence for a short period, it has already accumulated a great deal of experience. The difficulty with the Society of Authors is that technically you need to have published a book to be a member so that just when you most need advice it is not available; however, it is usually possible either to get unofficial help from the Medical Writers Group or, if you can show that you are in an advanced stage of negotiation about a nearly completed manuscript, to be admitted to associate membership. The latter is in itself an argument for taking your own work a good way down the line before starting to talk seriously to a publisher.

I shall now deal briefly with some matters which have proved important in some of the contracts I have been involved with:

Who has the copyright?

Publishers are much better able to defend copyright than you and though it may appear that you are sacrificing your independence it is usually better to vest it with them. Nevertheless, it is not necessary to sign away everything. Only "first serial rights in the UK and related English language export markets" is a good starting point. If then your book is a success you can make better terms for translations, student editions, etc. You should not believe however that you are very likely to make a lot of money from these—only rarely will this occur.

What about illustrations?

When I came into medical writing authors negotiated with artists and paid all the costs. Over the years artists have recognised that they are, like authors, relatively underpaid and that, in common with various segments of our own profession, they constitute a shortage speciality. Quite rightly they have increased their fees, so gobbling up a larger and larger proportion of the author's remuneration. Conclusions: illustrators should be employed by publishers and their fees be part of the book's production costs; some general agreement on the number of illustrations should be in the author's contract to safeguard both him and the publisher. It may well be that this will reduce your subsequent take home pay, but it is surprising how illustration costs have been absorbed into production costs over the last decade as publishers have had to be realistic. It is fair to say that most

247

(though not all) publishers recognise that authors should no longer pay for illustrations.

Index

Have nothing to do with it. Indices are professional matters and again should be part of the production costs. There is a strong cottage industry and you can indeed help your indexer to produce a good result (which will, of course, help your book) but do not take responsibility.

Incentive clauses

Try and negotiate a better deal to cover the event that the book sells better than anticipated.

Royalty versus down payment for contributors

Traditionally in a multiauthor text the editor gets royalties and contributors a one off down payment (contributors regard this as an editor getting rich while they lose money for the sake of doubtful prestige. Indeed it is less than ten years since I was asked to contribute a substantial segment of a well known text for the sole reward of a free copy *and* I had to pay for the illustrations). This scene must change and is changing, so that, as a few pioneering editors have already done, incentive repayments or better still royalties are paid to all. It is surprising what this can do to enhance loyalty to a book and that in the long run will help you with subsequent editions. The payment need not be so large as to whittle away all your own financial incentives.

Design

Do not, unless you are a real expert, meddle with design. Indeed it can be a plus point in your relations if you praise what the publisher does. He will usually be right and British book production still in my view leads the world.

Contributions

As a contributor with a subcontract to produce a portion of a book ask for payment not at publication but at the time of acceptance by the editor of your manuscript. This makes sure you do get paid for work done even if the book is not published.

Finally, one or two closing pieces of advice. At all stages resist

248

flattery. Publishers get most of their books by generating a false and immodest feeling that you, and you only, are the person who can write the most important, popular, scholarly, financially successful, immediately fame creating, and perpetually reissuable book on your chosen subject. Beware the bewitching horns of publishing faintly blowing because their thin clear notes are being produced many leagues away and the march to reach the reward they promise is a hard one. Unless you are a true and avowed mendicant scholar do keep the profit motive in mind. Dr Johnson's remark that no one but a fool writes except for money has been over quoted, but, like so much that self styled harmless drudge said, it has a tasty kernel of truth. Money is a great spur. There is quite a reasonable return for good writing and, properly managed in the UK at least, it can bestow significant tax advantages. Of course, one can make money faster and easier in private practice, on the stock exchange, or by farming but these comparisons are not exact for not all will find the pleasure in such pursuits as some of us will get from writing. So if we can profit in a modest way from our pleasure we should do so. Besides, the cut and thrust of negotiation with all those in publishing and books to achieve some reward brings one into contact with, in spite of my strictures, a body of men and women who, again in Johnson's words "are very clubbable." Of course, they rely on this fact and their company is so valuable that one forgets from time to time one's own advice; indeed I have written this contribution to a multiauthor book without a contract and for a flat fee. Stephen Lock has, as usual, outmanoeuvred me.

Review a book

HAROLD ELLIS

Even though I have done so myself on several occasions, I am always amazed that anyone ever succeeds in actually writing a book. To collect all the ideas and the facts first, then to put them down on paper in clear English, choose the illustrations and references, check them, and then to guide the whole lot through the intricacies of galley and page proofs, indexing, and tables of contents strike me as almost impossible tasks. And as for writing a novel or a play—they seem to me to be feats beyond human endeavour. Thus, when an editor asks me to review a book, my first thought is, "What a remarkable man this author must be to have got all this into print; he must be an extraordinarily knowledgeable and industrious fellow, and I doff my hat to him."

I feel I ought to make this confession (of which I am not the least bit ashamed) at the outset of this article because this accounts for the fact that I have the reputation of being a "kind reviewer." I suppose most people who have written books fall into the category, very much in the same way that a mother with six children is more likely to be sympathetic towards a girl in labour than a spinster or, worse still, a bachelor might be.

A duty to readers

I did my first medical book review 35 years ago and I suppose now I average about two dozen reviews a year. These are mostly of textbooks and monographs on general surgery, but also include volumes dealing with other specialities, including surgical anatomy and a few books of general medical interest or on paramedical subjects. Most of these I read right through fairly conscientiously, often as bedside reading, or late at night or at weekends. I admit that I only dip into the interesting parts of massive textbooks, read the new sections of further editions of those standard books that I already know fairly well, and I do *not* undertake to read medical dictionaries through from cover to cover. I read with a notebook alongside me so that I can jot down any comments as I go along, and I pay particular interest to the author's preface and to the "blurb" on the dustcover.

In preparing a review, I believe I have certain duties to perform on behalf of my readers. Firstly, I like to give some sort of background to the book's subject: is this of particular topical interest—for example, transplantation or the social aspects of mastectomy; does it fill a gap hitherto left open (I have just thought that there is no book entitled *Anatomy for Hospital Administrators*, and I will just make a note of that); or does it report on some important symposium (and, if so, how soon afterwards has the publisher got it on the market)? If possible, I then like to give some information about the author or authors, especially if I know them, and of their experience of the subject that they write about. Then I need to detail what the book contains, and to state whether or not it is readable, the print legible, illustrations relevant and suitably pictorial, and the bibliography reasonable and up to date.

After this, being a book lover, I consider whether it has that indefinable quality of being a book that it is a pleasure to own. Under this category are included such factors as the quality of the paper, binding, typography, and, of course, the smell. Finally, and very important indeed, I must state which members of the medical fraternity (if any) I will advise to puchase the commodity. On this I like to make up my mind. Reviewers are particularly allergic to dustcovers that state, "This important volume will prove invaluable to teaching hospital neurosurgeons, professors of urology, district hospital physicians, house surgeons, clinical and preclinical students, physiotherapists, and members of NUPE" unless, I suppose, it refers to the *Holy Bible*. In fact, with the degree of specialisation extant today, more and more books have appeal for smaller and smaller groups of specialist readers.

Constructive criticism only

I hardly ever mention the price of the book—unless to comment in those rare cases where it is surprisingly cheap. Being an unworldly academic, I do not think it is for me to argue with the publisher about the price he charges. Presumably he wishes to make his book as cheap as he possibly can compatible only with his making some sort of profit, because he knows that he can easily price himself out of the market. After all, I would rather have a first class book which I can own for ever than a first class meal, at the same price, whose pleasures are only transient and which is far less good for me. No, in my opinion, the price of the book is the concern of the purchaser and not the reviewer. It is he, and not I, who needs to decide whether or not he can afford it.

I also never enumerate a list of typographical errors in my reviews. I certainly state in no uncertain terms that a book is riddled with mistakes (usually associated with the related phenomenon of illustrations, especially x ray films, being upside down), and by and large such a book should be carefully avoided. If the authors have not checked the typography, they are equally likely to have been careless with their references and with the accuracy of their material. I do indeed make a note of any errors I come across (and I am sorry to say that careless proof reading and slack production are becoming yet another "English disease") and post the list to the authors. They are always grateful for such help and it is amazing how the same minor but annoying slip can go unnoticed in edition after edition of standard textbooks.

In my more depressed moments—usually when reviewing a book late at night—I naturally wonder whether the whole thing is really worth while; wouldn't it be better for journals to use their precious space for something else? When I cheer up again, however, I reassure myself that reviews of books, like those of films and plays, do have some important functions. Firstly, they act as a genuine guide to the purchaser, and I think many doctors decide whether or not to buy a book after reading one or two reviews about it. Speaking for myself, I buy medical books either because they are standard ones that I simply must possess for my work, or because they are written by friends of mine, or because I read about them in reviews and decide that they are for me. I am sure that many others follow these same guidelines. Secondly, reviews do act as a conscience and a quality control for our medical textbooks. A shoddy, badly written book will certainly receive its just punishment at the hands of even the kindest reviewers; a promising first edition will blossom out into a worthwhile revised version if the authors take cognisance of constructive review criticisms, and a world-beater will get to the public all the quicker when review readers realise this is something which must not be missed. Finally, and of this there is no doubt, book reviewing makes me read about 20 more books each year than I otherwise would, and for this I am duly grateful.

Beautify your old hospital

J H BARON

Why should hospitals be beautiful?

Sir Henry Wootton is usually remembered for defining an ambassador as "an honest man sent to lie abroad for the good of his country." But he equally pithily paraphrased Vitruvius's qualities of a building (strength/utility/beauty), "Well building hath three conditions, commoditie, firmenes and delight."[1] A hospital is designed to work as a health care factory, and does so more or less effectively. Not all contemporary hospitals fall down, from lapses of design and execution, soon after they are completed. But how few expect their hospital to be designed and built for delight. I find it curious that those who like their home to be elegant, who museum crawl and sightsee on holiday at home and abroad, are amazed when I suggest that a hospital should be beautiful, and provide a life enhancing experience for staff, patients, and visitors.

It is only during the last half of this century that my ambitions are considered eccentric. No one thought it odd that Hogarth should have painted murals at Bart's. The Victorians expected their town halls and railway stations to be objects of wonder and beauty; the walls of some of their children's wards were covered with fairy tales and nursery rhymes in Doulton tiles; even a workhouse might have pictures on the walls (fig 1). Those who trained at Middlesex will remember its elegant panelled front hall, with Cayley Robinson's *Acts of Mercy* murals, the central circular table with the daily change of flowers, the brass-buttoned, frock-coated uniformed porters, and the singular lettering of the ward names on the direction boards. Think of most hospital entrances today.

If you accept my premise then this chapter will help you to beautify your old hospital. If you want your new hospital to have works of art you may find ideas in a separate article.[2]

253

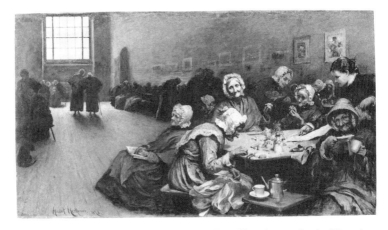

Fig 1—*Sir H van Herkomer (1849–1914). Eventide—A scene in the Westminster Union, 1878 Walker Art Gallery, Liverpool.*

Apathy and antipathy

Do not be put off by lack of interest. Achievement is still possible in the face of amused tolerance so long as you press on regardless.

Although apathy can be brushed aside, actual anatagonism will stop you. You will fail if you meet explicit opposition from any power figure. I made hints at two hospitals world famous for their clinical science. In one, "The sad facts are, even in periods of financial boom, no one would consider art as a necessary portion of hospital expenditure." In the other the dean did consult his advisory committee and heads of department: "There wasn't a very enthusiastic response. Perhaps we are all a bit overwhelmed with the general gloom, particularly on the NHS side. . . ." Faced with these reactions, give up and wait for a new dean, who is "interested in changing what is unquestionably one of the most squalid hospitals in all Britain."

The committee

In any facet of British public life, and especially in a hospital within a bureaucratic health service, you need a committee for any new venture to succeed. Some hospitals use conventional names, an art or arts committee, a fine arts board, a history and works of art committee: I was forthright and called ours the beautification committee. You need terms of reference which should be as wide as your interests. You must report to someone, such as the unit

254

management team of a hospital, or the special trustees if they are the prime paymaster.

The other reason for a committee is to spread the aesthetic responsibility. The directors of the National Gallery and the Tate may buy nothing on their own decisions: the trustees have to approve every purchase, so that the responsibility for acts of expenditure of public money can be spread among, and any obloquy borne by, many broad shoulders. Similarly, in a hospital there will be strong criticism of anything you do: let it it be clear that decisions have been shared and conclusions reached by thoughtful people.

The committee must be small and meet regularly on a specific day and time. If you are chairman you need an interested administrator, interested nursing officer, and the key figure, the committee secretary, who must have a devotion to the topic, and can come from any discipline—for example, the voluntary services organiser if you have one, or an outside art lover in an honorary capacity.

What to beautify

Buildings

Every hospital was designed by an architect with skill, devotion, and artistry. Often the original drawings or engravings survive or can be found in illustrations in old books, local newspapers, the topography collection of your library, architectural journals, or national periodicals such as the *Illustrated London News*. These designs will grace an entrance hall or corridor, framed as pictures or as black and white photographic enlargements blown up to whole wall size.

All too many British hospitals were built a century ago as Victorian workhouse infirmaries for the sick poor. The nineteenth century buildings have usually been altered, or extensions of every style added, leaving a mish mash of an architectural jungle. But sometimes the original buildings have not been so disturbed. If you can persuade the works department to remove decades of grime you may be pleasantly surprised at the splendours of Victorian brickwork, detailings, and architecture. You may find your principal work of art is your own building. If so, cherish it. See that there is an overall colour scheme for the exterior wood work and drainpipes, that the roofing is repaired in colour and texture similar to the original: if you cannot afford new real slates at least have simulated ones. If there are original iron railings, fences, balconies, or walkways try to keep them and prevent their replacement by barbed wire or chicken fencing. Similarly, the original lamps may have been gas lit and can be adapted to electricity rather than replaced by concrete posts.

In lieu of a brand new hospital you will probably be given new additions for outpatient or x ray departments: if you are not careful some prefabricated concrete box will rise up and mar the old ensemble. Try to persuade your district to set up a design panel which must see and approve aesthetically, and not just functionally, all new additions to any hospital in the district, so that representations can be made before it is too late and the juggernaut of the NHS planning process rolls over you.

Gardens

These are best left to garden experts, one or two of whom are bound to be found in your committee or can be co-opted. Your garden subgroup should take a look at the whole hospital campus and make recommendations via your committee to the unit management team about the outside lawns, trees, paved areas, benches, tubs, climbers and plants, ponds and fountains, not to forget litter bins. There may be scope for some indoor plant schemes, but every scheme must be manageable either by named and interested volunteers from staff or friends, or by contract with a garden firm.

Hospital entrances

These come in all sizes and shapes, but are rarely welcoming. The casualty department is often approached through a tiled tunnel or corridor lined with wheelchairs. The outpatient department may be hidden down a side street and the waiting hall filled with broken chairs, tattered magazines, blaring television, ashtrays, and countless notices, hortatory or admonitory, ranging from injunctions to tell the desk if you have changed you name or your family doctor to warnings about smoking, drinking, and the problems and consequences of life after sex.

Most visitors come into a main courtyard and are immediately made unwelcome by a kaleidoscope of notices forbidding them to park (reserved for consultants), or warning that they park at their own risk, or telling them how to get to the special clinic or the mortuary.

Inside, the main hall is cluttered with more notices, telephone boothes, fire extinguishers, post boxes, flower stalls, newspaper kiosks, and sometimes a reception desk with pigeon holes for letters, fuseboxes, and a keyboard. A sympathetic architect should be commissioned to design a comprehensive plan for refurbishing, lighting, and decorating your front hall. He may be able to bring the porters' desk forward and flank it with a general shop and a flower stall with telephone alcoves at each end. The clutter of objects and notices can be removed and tidied up visually. It is often helpful to lower the ceiling, install concealed lighting and bank the direction signs into blocks of colours to complement the whole colour scheme.

Notices

These spring up everywhere and can mostly be removed. A map is ideal with a plan of the hospital or even a model. Obviously directions are needed to the different wards and departments. Most hospitals have been persuaded by the DHSS to use their standardised lower case sans serif typeface for every sign. Some people like it. It is a matter of taste. Such lettering is ideal for motorway signs for clarity and ease of reading as you rush past in your car. I am depressed by seeing the same institutional lettering in every hospital. It may suit hospitals that look like motorways. For your hospital, look at other typefaces in in the catalogues of notice makers—perhaps Times New Roman will suit your own buildings best.

Ideally your hospital, and indeed your district, should have a corporate image, with a logo and an elegant type face for everything it presents to the public, whether on the flags flying overhead, the names on the vans going through the streets, the signs over the entrance, the writing paper and the mail franking.

Corridors

Until recently most district and many university hospitals were designed on the Nightingale pattern, a long corridor off which branched several two or three storey ward blocks. This design allowed natural light and ventilation to enter the wards from two sides, and separate each ward from another by a distance sufficient to lessen crossinfection and noise. Another happy consequence of this design is that staff meet each other walking up and down the corridors, and do not spend their time in isolation waiting for, or crowded into, the lifts of the vertically designed hospitals of today.

However, long main corridors are often the most aesthetically depressing part of a British hospital. The visitor's heart sinks as he sees a gloomy prospect with the end scarcely in view, frequently in a grubby decorative state, or, even when freshly painted, in a

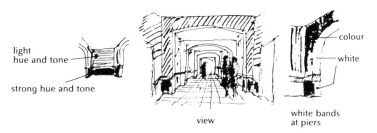

Fig 2—*Corridor colour scheme by Robert Radford, 1984. The objective is to provide a linking line of colour to the chair rail and a sequence of hues to each bay emphasised by the strong hues below the chair rail punctuated by white elements.*

drab single colour.[3] Ask your architect to consider breaking the corridor into different coloured areas. He may want to coordinate and to classify his colour on some such scheme as the Munsell system, and then give you a linking line of colour with a sequence of hues to each bay (fig 2).

How to beautify

Murals

You may have an entrance stairway or foyer, or a busy corridor leasing to outpatients. These can be key areas visually and cry out for murals. They are places of continual movement, where it is perhaps undesirable for people to stop, stand, and scrutinise recognisable representational objects in a mural. Perhaps an abstract pattern could be used to better advantage. The mural must work as a simple immediate effect unfolding as the visitor walks past, and by its optimism relieve the tension of those who are worrying about themselves or others. In other departments, such as a visitors waiting area, or for those sitting in chairs or lying on stretchers (for example, outside radiotherapy) pastoral scenes or flowers may be more restful. Day areas might be cheered by local topography, past or present. The needs of children's units are obvious.

Pictures

These can adorn most walls, but need to be chosen for size and colour for a specific site. They are particularly needed in long corridors, in waiting areas. in day rooms, and in foyers outside wards. Persuade your colleagues to donate, or at least pay for, framed photographs of the notable who gives his name to their wards (Addison, Fleming, Churchill, etc). You may be asked for pictures for individual offices, in which case you should have an operational policy that pictures are provided from hospital funds only for public spaces—that is, where the public walks and in offices where patients or visitors come: other office holders should certainly be encouraged to have pictures—their own.

Hospital wards have surprisingly little space for pictures, usually only a few walls are sufficiently bare for hanging because most walls in a ward are taken up with windows, cupboards, or have wires trailing and tubes attached. Even in sidewards you should be careful not to trap a patient face to face with an incompatible picture for days or weeks on end.

Conservation

Pictures cannot be left to look after themselves any more than laws can be left to enforce themselves. An institution should not buy, and certainly not borrow, works of art unless it is prepared to catalogue, conserve, and generally keep an eye on them to prevent loss and damage. This task should be assigned to one interested and obsessional individual, who could be an expert volunteer or from the administrative, nursing, or paramedical staff.

If you do borrow from public bodies you will have to insure the work at their valuation: few hospitals have either the time or expertise to deal with such administrative problems. For example, in 1965 the Walker Art Gallery lent pictures which were hung in the entrance hall of the Liverpool Royal Infirmary: the security arrangements were later considered inadequate and the gallery withdrew its pictures.[4] Pictures continually disappear from hospitals. Theft is probably rare: more often the pictures are taken down and not properly stored when a ward or corridor is to be cleaned. When the decorations are completed the pictures are not rehung, they are mislaid, discarded, or lost. The donor who in 1912 gave tens of thousands of pounds to each of at least eight hospitals to bear the name of his widow Annie Zunz also gave a portrait to hang in the ward. Who can find Annie Zunz today?[5]

Anything hanging on a hook can all to easily be carried off. The pictures need to be fixed firmly to a wall by screws—with mirror plates, for example. If the hospital engineers cannot spare appropriate staff for this task then professional picture hangers will be needed. The pictures must not be exposed to intense light or heat, wind, rain or humidity.

All pictures need framing, and all watercolours and engravings and some paintings need glazing too. Works on paper need mounting on acid free boards. Even a large occupational therapy department is unlikely to be able to cope with such requirements, and professional framers should be used, with thoughtful and individual consideration of the type of mount and frame suitable for each work.

Pictures need labels to tell the viewer at least the title and the artist. These are best pinned to the lower horizontal of the frame and the size, colour and lettering will depend on the colour and texture of the picture mount and frame, and again is usually best done professionally. Large works such as murals deserve a large wall mounted label giving not only title, artist, and date but also the occasion of its commissioning and the donors; a few lines explaining the composition may be helpful too.

Quite apart from the simple labels you need a card index, detailing for each object the artist, with date of birth (and where appropriate death), the date and title of the composition, the medium (oil, watercolour, engraving, etching) and the material (canvas, board, paper, etc), the date of purchase, the cost and source of funds (or from whom borrowed and when and for how long), and its location. Some of these data can be turned into a catalogue which can be duplicated or printed according to your resources.

Finance

The old board of governors voluntary hospitals all had endowment funds which have been preserved in the care of special trustees. You may be able to persuade them that they should spend some of their income, or even their capital, on works of art. Some have allotted tens of thousands of pounds for initial purchases, and then provided up to £10 000 a year for staff, further purchases, and conservation. Others spend nothing on art.

If your special trustees refuse you money for works of art, or you are in an old municipal county council hospital without special trustees, you may find your district has some free money, their share of the old area health authority's trust funds. Your unit too may have some free money from donations or legacies from grateful patients and well wishers. Funds may be raised by friends or volunteers, especially for specific purposes like pictures for a refurbished day room.

Study some of the available booklets[6-10] for ideas on funding and names and addresses.[8,11] Discuss your requirements with the visual arts officer of your regional arts association and the director of your local art gallery. In London the Public Art Development Trust will tell you about the Greater London Arts

260

Association/King's Fund mural scheme. The Manpower Services Commission may help you with a project for training the unemployed, as craftsmen in the arts, or you can approach local industry, and national foundations. Pictures can be borrowed from Paintings in Hospitals and prints from the British Red Cross Society.

You will probably be wise to avoid, even if you are able to obtain, exchequer funds from the hospital budget. You can steel yourself against criticisms of your aesthetic judgment and taste in any beautification you promote. However, if there was any payment for a work of art you may find "the correspondence columns of the local newspaper immediately filled up with letters from Mr Disgusted Taxpayer (who else?)—a man who didn't know anything about art, but knew what he disliked. If this money had not been wasted on so-called modern art my grannie could have had her teeth taken out and a new gas stove put in."[12]

The visit

The NHS, like all great institutions, has an inertia of its own which will stop all your initiatives from starting, and prevent the completion of any which began. You may speed up your project by the usual wheedling and negotiations, but faced with an impasse play your ace, the visit. Arrange for some dignitary (be it royalty, the regional chairman, or the mayor) to come on a specific date to open one of your schemes and unveil an appropriately worded plaque in the presence of an invited audience. You will be pleasantly surprised how the impossible begins to happen at once, that timetables of work are kept, and that the hospital, or at least the professional route of the tour by the visitor, has been cleaned.

Conclusion

Now that you have read this article do you still want to beautify your hospital? You can do so, just as you can achieve anything else in the health service given vision, energy, time and patience, a lack of enemies, a working committee, and sufficient guile to know both the regulations which run the NHS and how to outwit them.

Many have helped and are thanked elsewhere.[6] In this endeavour, as in so much else, I was inspired by my wife.

[1] Wootton H. *Elements of architecture.* London: John Bill, 1624: 1.
[2] Baron J H, Greene L. Funding works of art in new hospitals. *Br Med J* 1984; **289**: (in press).
[3] Agate J. Colour in hospitals. *World Medicine* 1969; 20 May: 13–7.

[4] Brewer C. *Liverpool Royal Infirmary, 1887–1978*. Liverpool: Area Health Authority (Teaching), 1980, 131.

[5] Rosse E M. The lady missing from St Mary's. *Nor West*, 1984, **2**, (3): 2.

[6] Baron J H, Hadden M. *St Charles Hospital works of art*. London, 1984.

[7] Coles P. *The Manchester Hospital Arts Project*. London: Calouste Gulbenkian Foundation, 1981.

[8] Coles P. *Art in the National Health Service. A report by the DHSS*. London: DHSS, 1983. (Obtainable Rm 502, 286 Euston Rd, London NW1.)

[9] Hyslop R. *Art in hospitals. Conference Report*. London DHSS, 1983.

[10] Reed E. Art in hospitals. *Arts Review*, 1983, 13 May: 259.

[11] Townsend P, ed. *Art within reach: artists and craftworkers, architects and patrons in the making of public art*. London: Art Monthly/Thames and Hudson, 1984.

[12] Keep P. Having an art attack. *World Medicine*, 1983, 25 June: 22.

Fly

IAN CAPPERAULD

There is only one way to fly and that is first class. However, not all of us can afford to fly first class and it should be remembered that first class treatment stops when you reach your destination and starts only when you reach the airport. The object of this paper is to give a few practical hints on how to fly in the most comfortable fashion prepared for all eventualities no matter whether you are flying Concorde, first class, "tourist," or Super Apex.

Preparation for the journey

It is not my intention to tell you how to pack or what to pack but there are certain points which must be remembered.

(1) Do not put a copy of your lecture or slides in the hold baggage. Carry them with you.

(2) Carry a spare bag in your suitcase to bring back literature and goods you have purchased since they will not cram into your hold baggage.

(3) Carry a spare string carrier bag with you which will accommodate your duty free on the way out and your duty free on the way back. The string bag is not so inclined to give way as are the normal plastic bags given away at duty free shops.

(4) Carry a briefcase. Ideally it should contain the following articles:

- A wallet specially fitted with compartments to carry your passport, airline tickets, travellers cheques, boarding card, receipts, vaccination certificates, and any other documents which you may require for the journey. (Keep your luggage tags separate rather than being affixed to the ticket.)
- A screwdriver, or preferably a Swiss Army knife, which will allow you to change plugs in your hotel room. It is impossible to carry all types of adapters, but taking one plug off a lamp in the

263

room and fixing it to your own electrical gadget will enable you to use this equipment.

- Have a pen which enables you to fill in your landing card. People usually leave their pens in their jackets which are hung up and there is a scramble at the time of landing to fill in the landing form. Incidentally, always make a point of completing the landing form immediately you receive it. This is in case you are unable to complete it coherently because of liberal supplies of alcohol.
- Carry dollars in single dollar notes as these are invaluable for porters and to obtain taxis even in Communist bloc countries.
- A shoehorn is invaluable to put your own shoes on following a long flight. You will find that this is also more than useful to your travelling companions.
- A shaving kit which allows you to arrive fresh at your destination.
- A clean shirt which will allow you to change before landing and allow you to arrive fresh.

Incidentally, both the shaving kit and shirt become invaluable in the event that you are diverted to another destination without access to baggage in the hold.

Most of the above items apply also to women who are travelling except that the appropriate clothing and perhaps cosmetics should be substituted so that they feel fresh on arrival.

(5) Medicines: At an early point in the preparation for the journey a decision has to be made, since you are a doctor, about the medicines you take with you. The decision is that of taking medicines to treat yourself or taking medicines to treat any or many of your travelling companions. Because of the implications of international laws and the areas over which you are flying, I personally restrict the medicines I take for myself. Some of the medicines can be carried in your briefcase and others in the hold baggage.

Certainly, it pays to carry aspirin or paracetamol and, if you have difficulty in sleeping on an overnight flight, some form of hypnotic such as Mogadon. Other medicines which are particularly useful are listed:

Avomine	Travel sickness
Imodium	Diarrhoea
Maxolon	Nausea or sickness in gastroenteritis
Fabahistin	Allergic conditions
Paludrine	
Maloprim	Antimalarial
Chloroquine	

| Septrin | Urinary infections |
| Tetracycline | Respiratory infections |

Although essentially not forming part of a medical kit as such, I find it useful to carry the following in the hold baggage, which can make life bearable in otherwise adverse conditions.

- A solid rubber ball which will act as a bath plug or a sink plug.
- Soap.
- Toilet paper.
- Insect repellant and room freshener spray.
- Presept tablets, which are a form of sodium hypochloride or bleach and which are invaluable for putting down the toilet or bath in hotels where the plumbing and the cleaning leaves a lot to be desired.

At the airport

Determine whether the plane is going to take off on time and, if it is not, the alternatives for rerouting to get to your destination at the time you want to be there. There are warning signs of impending delay such as the flight number not appearing on the board and if the announcement detailing the delay is "indefinitely" this can often be interpreted as at least a six hour delay.

When reserving your seat try to get one beside an emergency exit which, apart from giving you an element of safety, also gives you an element of comfort since by law the space at the emergency door is always 50% greater than in the rest of the plane.

Buying duty free is not always now a bargain or even necessary since in countries like America alcohol is usually cheaper, and in countries like Russia and Poland there are duty free shops in which you can buy any form of alcohol by using hard currency and at a rate cheaper than at the airport. However, the purchase of cigarettes for friends is often well received, especially in those countries where only local brands are sold.

While it may be tempting to have cups of coffee or alcohol before boarding the plane, there is usually a queue after take off for toilet facilities and, therefore, it is better to restrict your intake.

On board the plane

There is a lot of advice written on how to fly in comfort and indeed many exercises which can be performed do help to pass the time or to prevent deep vein thrombosis. One of the best ways of relieving boredom and of trying to prevent deep vein thrombosis is to make an active effort to get up out of your seat and wander round the plane. To this end, therefore, you will be less of a nuisance to your travelling companions if you choose an aisle seat rather than a window seat. If you are not fortunate enough to travel first class where slipperettes are provided, carry an extra pair of socks or obtain a pair of slipperettes to put on your feet since no matter how fit you are or whatever your age group, inevitably some form of gravitation oedema does occur when sitting for long periods. Walking around the plane also helps to dispel the effects of sitting. If you are flying from west to east overnight and, because of the time lag, you will be arriving at your destination early in the morning but it will still be late in the evening at your point of departure, it is extremely important that you do not have an excess of food or alcohol on that journey. Going through customs and immigration tired is one thing but bloated and merry is another.

Arrival

Get a porter. It is money well spent since he will get you a trolley, get you through customs, and get you a taxi. When considering what to pay for this service always pay \$1 per piece of luggage carried and you will not go far wrong. If you are in any doubt as to whether you are being charged properly or overcharged by the taxi driver get him to carry your luggage into the hotel or indeed get the hotel to pay the taxi for you and put it on to the bill, especially if you have not changed money into the local currency. If possible, change your money at the bank rather than the hotel as there is usually a charge of $7\frac{1}{2}$–10% levied by the hotel for changing currency.

Conclusions

Flying can be fun but arriving at your destination safe, fresh, and comfortable, knowing that your slides and your lectures are with you, and that you are prepared for all eventualities, be it friend or foe, can be a comfort and a consolation and, as I said at the beginning, first class treatment stops frequently when you arrive at your destination.

266